195

You Can Be

Physically Perfect, Powerfully Strong

You Can Be
Physically Perfect, Powerfully Strong

Vic Boff

ARCO PUBLISHING COMPANY, INC.
219 Park Avenue South, New York, N.Y. 10003

Published by Arco Publishing Company, Inc.
219 Park Avenue South, New York, N.Y. 10003

Library of Congress Catalog Card Number 74-82866

ISBN 0-668-02700-2

Printed in the United States of America

*Dedicated
to the late
Bernarr Macfadden
and
George F. Jowett
who inspired my
early physical
culture life*

Contents

Physical Fitness, Life's Greatest Asset   1
Developing Organic Health   4
Train Yourself to Breathe   8
Proper Posture Is a Vital Necessity   14
Basic Foundation Conditioning   19
Treasure Your Chest   52
Trim Your Waistline   68
Put Power into Your Legs   86
Strong Bodies Need Strong Spines   110
Why You Should Have a Strong Neck   129
You, Too, Can Build Strong Arms   145
Put Some Stretch into Your
     Muscle-Building Program   166
Keep Your Feet Healthy and Happy   172
Know Your Muscles   175
Food, Diet, and the Health Builder   180
Sleep   199
Sun Baths   200
Get Outdoors and Live   202
Use Your Time Wisely for Bodybuilding
     Success   206
The Tools for Physical Fitness   210
Index   213

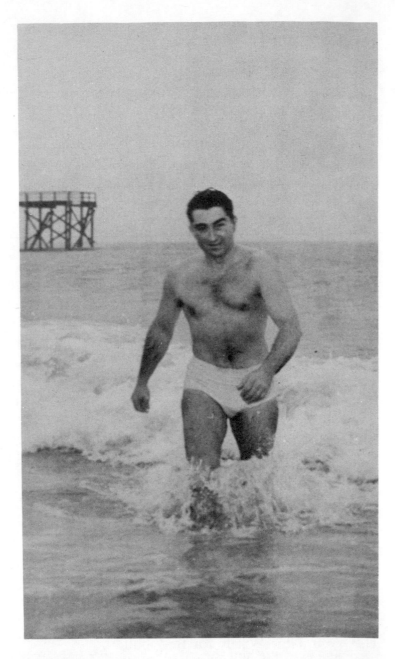

Vic Boff is an ardent year-round outdoor man. Here he comes
dashing out of the surf at Coney Island in the middle of winter.

Physical Fitness, Life's Greatest Asset

The magnificent human specimens of ancient Greece were not God-created; they were the result of systematic physical training. Regular exercise was as much a part of their lives as eating and sleeping, because they recognized that harmonious development of all parts of the body was essential to good health. History tells us how truly great these people were—as long as they remained faithful to their ideals.

Many people are concerned with the problem of physical fitness in today's society. Modern living conditions have caused the average person to become flabby and physically inefficient. The great majority have relegated themselves to the role of spectators while watching a proportionately few athletes pursue their activities. This "spectator tendency," combined with health-depleting indoor occupations, has caused ill health, weakness, and premature aging.

In every human being today there is the potential for developing as much health, strength, and beauty as there was in the days of the ancient Greeks. Skeptics speak contemptuously of those following the physical culture life; they feel that they are alive and healthy because they can get out of bed, walk around, and perform the day's tasks. No greater delusion can exist about the proper functioning of the human body. Real health and strength means unlimited vitality. It means exuberant spirits and a capacity for endless work. It insures an active, clear mind and a pleasing personality. It allows one to realize all his possibilities. These attributes become a reality when all-around physical movements are applied to the body in a way compatible with the modern way of life.

There are over five hundred muscles in the human body, and these make up nearly one-half of our bodily bulk. The vital functions of the internal organs are profoundly affected by the condition of these muscles. Their proper action and coordination is essential to the regulation of the life processes. Health associates itself with internal as well as external strength. Whenever health is impaired, strength decreases; therefore, health and strength are inseparable. The balance between them is maintained by proper exercise, which is a necessary muscular activity.

Appropriate exercise provides a means to regenerate the entire organism. It increases the absorption of oxygen in the body, produces vigorous circulation, strengthens the heart and blood vessels, and speeds up elimination. It is nature's weapon against physical deficiency and ill health. The intelligent application of exercise will bring wonderful results in restoring health and in the correction of many physical deformities. It is the governing factor in the entire health scheme, which also includes other hygienic factors such as a good diet, fresh air and sun baths, relaxation and the necessary amount of sleep, etc., all determined by individual needs.

Puny, skinny, undernourished youths have been transformed into powerful, radiantly healthy men with beautiful bodies by simple, pleasant, home methods of bodybuilding exercises. It is within everyone's power to have a better physique. True, a fine physique may be denied to a few because of heredity or disease. However, there is not one man, woman, or child in this world who, provided he has the will and the desire and is free from organic disease, cannot improve his body beyond all expectations by following a sensible program of progressive exercises.

I do not wish to give the impression that you have to become an athlete or strong man to acquire physical fitness, but rather to emphasize the necessity of activity for bodily health.

Exercise which is performed regularly, judiciously, and in graduated amounts will give you a greater sense of well-being and increase your capacity to enjoy life to the fullest. Your physical appearance will be improved. You will eat and sleep better and will be able to work with zest and enthusiasm; life will be more enjoyable. In short, physical fitness will give you a healthy body that is strong, beautiful, and radiant with energy.

Developing Organic Health

The Inner Man Comes First

You can't build muscles unless your internal organs are in good condition. The degree of your organic health is the yardstick by which you can measure your bodybuilding possibilities. If your organic tone is low, no material physical improvement will take place until you put your internal house in order. The best slogan for you to remember is: "Build from the inside out."

Bodily energy is created by the chemistry of the internal organs. This chemistry supplies the nutritive fuel for building the cellular muscular structure, is the source of strength, the basis of vitality, and the foundation of bodily endurance. All of which should tell you that you cannot expect to develop a healthy, well-muscled, powerful body unless your internal organs are functioning efficiently.

Why some bodybuilders fail

Unfortunately, I often see aspiring bodybuilders striving to develop their muscles at the expense of their organs, with the result that they fail to achieve their goal. They never learned the simple fact that *you cannot build your muscles at the sacrifice of your organic health.* Nature will not let you! You must build from the inside out, and when you do, your success in reaching physical perfection will be assured.

Because of this, every beginner should arrange his

4

training on a graduated scale. The first few weeks of training should be devoted to toning the internal organs. From then on, the exercises should be those which efficiently maintain a balance between the organs and the muscles.

If this progressive method is followed, the balance of power will always rest with the organs. This is sensible, because it means that no matter how powerfully the body is built, organic secretion will be available in abundance to protect and fortify the muscular system against harm. This balance can be readily detected. By nature, the muscles tire first. When this happens, the organic forces are unaffected, and are able to function freely for rapid physical recuperation.

Toning is not a waste of time

Some bodybuilders object to spending the time to tone their internal organs. They think that the exercises provided for toning are too simple because they do not require the vigorous effort expended in exercises designed for strong muscular action. They should remember that you cannot force *organic* improvement, as is possible with the muscles. The organs respond only to persuasion, and these exercises can be as interesting as they are stimulating.

Exercise stimulates the organic processes, and as long as the heart, lungs, and digestive and excretory organs can meet the demands of a vigorously active system, the whole system benefits by the increased exercise. The body develops best during growth periods if the brain and muscles are exercised to the limit of their powers so that the system as a whole responds to their organic demands. To achieve full development of every power, unrelenting activity is necessary from the cradle onward.

Calisthenics are not used for organic toning. The

exercise movements should be a combination of muscular and respiratory; neither deep breathing nor freehand movements are sufficient alone. Only a combination concentrating on both the chest and the abdominal region will be effective. These exercises must be stepped up daily, and slowly changed to those of a more advanced order. Progress should be gradual and scientific.

After a month on this toning program, the novice can begin more vigorous exercises. His former training will have fortified him and accustomed him to the right method of breathing with each new exercise, so that he can perform every movement automatically and maintain a harmonious rhythm between the respiratory and the muscular systems. This will develop the natural balance that builds reservoirs of energy to nourish and fertilize the growing muscles.

Natural methods are best

By following this natural order, both muscle tissue and strength are developed quickly, and a foundation of organic endurance is laid at the same time. For this reason, modern progressive courses of bodybuilding based on this logical method take the pupil, step by step, from one stage of development to another until he becomes capable of performing the most vigorous exercises with an ease and efficiency not possible with unbalanced training programs.

No apparatus is needed for this form of training but your own body weight. Do not get the idea that this is easy, or that the exercises are easy. Many of them will tax the strength of the strongest man for no other reason than that at all times he is handling part, or all, of his own body weight, using the muscles in their proper capacity as natural levers to supply the strength to lift his body. This is the natural way.

Strength that lasts

Once the bodily systems, both muscular and organic, have reached a natural high level, then, and only then, is the beginner ready to enter the field of strenuous exercise. By this time his body will be splendidly developed with proportionate strength.

Those who are sensible enough to build their bodily health and strength on these foundations build for life. According to the natural law of life, middle age should be full of youthful vigor.

A man should be at his best in his forties and into his sixties, as the vast strength he has acquired in his youth becomes matured in what we term the middle years. Records prove that some of the greatest strength records were performed by men in their forties and fifties. John Y. Smith, of Boston, defeated the cream of the American weight lifters in an open contest at the age of sixty years and sixty-six days. This is not an unusual case; history is full of such achievements.

The answer to the search for lasting strength and a durable muscular body lies in placing *organic* health first. The organs can then take care of the muscles and help to develop a powerful, symmetrical body.

Train Yourself to Breathe

Breathing is the vital force of life. The human body can go without food for weeks and without water for days—but check the free flow of air to the lungs for a few seconds and death will result. Nothing else absorbed by the body, whether food, water, or any other substance required to sustain life, is as necessary as air. Air is to the human body what a draft is to a furnace: cut off the draft—oxygen—and you will kill the fire, no matter what quality or quantity of coal you use. Cut off the free supply of oxygen to your lungs through shallow breathing and your blood will become impoverished and poisoned, no matter what quality or quantity of food you eat. The faster you run, the faster you must breathe. The more intensely you think, the more oxygen you consume. Every act of the human body, from winking an eyelid to lifting enormous weights, requires the consumption of oxygen, which can only be replaced in one way: by breathing. Every nervous impulse and every pulsation of the heart means that a certain amount of fuel has been consumed, and this process leaves a deadly poison in the blood—carbon dioxide. Carbon dioxide is so deadly that if it is permitted to accumulate and remain in the blood for only a few seconds, every cell in the body becomes mortally infected, and immediate death is the result. It is the duty of the lungs to free the blood of this poison. As it circulates through the lungs, the dark venous blood exchanges carbon dioxide for life-giving oxygen. Thus the lungs perform a great double duty—they oxygenate the blood and also purify it.

8

Your lungs are your respiratory organs, through which oxygen is absorbed to permeate your entire system. It is also your lungs that expel the greatest quantity of carbon dioxide through exhalation. Offhand, you would say that breathing exercise is your remedy. It is and it is not. If you do not understand the processes of the lungs—how they function in oxygen distribution, and get rid of carbon dioxide—your efforts may be fruitless. You must first ascertain the condition of your respiratory system.

Do you use only one-fifth of your lung powers?

The average person only employs about one-fifth of his lung capacity. Normally, you have a breathing capacity of 230 to 250 cubic inches, depending upon your age and weight. Your lungs are composed of multitudinous air chambers, through the walls of which oxygen is passed into the blood stream. The intake of air is not just a simple thing like gulping in the air with a deep breath, and then leaving it to permeate the air chambers. The air in your lungs is divided into several components, known as the complemental, supplemental, and residual, and certain amounts of permeation and exchange take place in each. The most important of the three is the residual, which is the deepest-seated air circulatory environment. The quantity of air here never changes. The air remains and, as the name "residual" indicates, it is resident there. It is impossible to exhaust this part of the air in your lungs, and foolish to think you can, or to try to empty your lungs, as so many advocate, in breathing out. The important exchange between oxygen and waste gas or carbon dioxide takes place in the residual system. This exchange is made through your capillary system, a fine network of tiny blood vessels.

The fact that only one-fifth of your breathing system is used naturally means that a considerable portion of your lungs is in an unused condition, and is probably clogged with waste. You should no more think of expecting to use your lungs to their fullest capacity at the beginning of your exercise program than you would dream of expecting to use a machine efficiently without first cleaning away the corrosive dirt. It is logical to assume that you should approach the conditioning of your respiratory system in the same way. Care is needed because the cell walls in the lungs are constructed of delicate membranes which can be easily ruptured. The whole work of toning your lungs is not done by the act of deep breathing alone; your internal and external muscular systems must also be considered.

Why the usual popular methods of deep breathing are dangerous to your health

It was once popular to simply practice deep breathing for the lungs, with the result that the lungs were capable of a voluminous intake and expiration under conscious action. However, when the conscious exercise was stopped, and one reverted to the natural, autonomous act of breathing, the amount of air absorbed was as small as before one took up the practice. This is due to the fact that the internal muscles had not been developed, and neither had the external muscles. Your lungs are encased in a bony cage we call the chest box. If your muscles are underdeveloped or emaciated from neglect, your chest box is smaller than normal, and your lungs do not have much natural space to expand in, except when you consciously force them to do so. The internal muscles attached to the inside of your ribs and surrounding your lungs provide the strength to expand your lungs. These muscles are constantly exerting their pressure against your lungs, and then relaxing. Consequently, you can see why deep breathing alone is a waste of time.

Expansion is muscular

Expansion of the rib box, which dilates the lungs, is carried out entirely by muscular action. The chest is enlarged from back to front and from side to side by the action of the intercostal and other auxiliary muscles of respiration, and from top to bottom by the action of the diaphragm, a muscle whose action is almost entirely involuntary.

The structure of the thorax and lungs is such that unless the chest is enlarged in all three directions air cannot penetrate to all of the millions of air sacs in the lungs. Diaphragmatic breathing, which some maintain is the correct way to breathe, aerates only the lower air sacs of the lungs. Costal breathing aerates only the middle and upper parts. Without a doubt, the correct way to breathe is to use a combination of both methods.

Most people, particularly sedentary workers, are "shallow breathers," breathing at an average rate of from 17 to 20 times per minute, and only taking in about ten percent of what is, or should be, their total lung capacity with each breath. The inevitable result of shallow breathing, if it is allowed to become a habit, is that when an occasion arises for the breathing apparatus to be used to full capacity, it breaks down, and the individual gets winded or "short of breath" and suffers acute distress. What has happened is that the respiratory muscles have been allowed to get weak and flabby through lack of use and neglect, and cannot respond to an unaccustomed call upon them, while the lung tissues themselves have lost some of their resiliency.

The remedy for this situation is to develop the habit of taking much more air into the lungs with each breath; in other words, to breathe deeply, using costal as well as diaphragmatic breathing, and to breathe fewer times per minute. This does not necessarily mean that a greater quantity of air (and consequently of oxygen) is used per minute, but it does mean that the whole breathing mechanism is used more thoroughly, the muscles which operate it can develop properly, the costal cartilages retain their elasticity and the lung tissues their resiliency, and all parts of the lungs are properly aerated. This last point is important: in shallow breathing a large proportion of the carbon dioxide carried to the lungs reaches air sacs which are never dilated, and therefore it is not expelled and is returned by the pulmonary circulatory system to the heart, and from there into the general circulatory system, where it acts as a poison.

Another very important aspect which follows from the cultivation of the habit of deep breathing is that not only the respiratory muscles but also those of the shoulders, abdomen, back, and arms develop more rapidly. No pair of lungs has ever been damaged by deep breathing, yet no other part of the human body is more liable to suffer damage and disease through neglect and nonuse.

The object is to build all these muscles, both internal and external, in proportion to the improved condition of your lungs, in which case your internal muscles are vigorously active. In developing your external chest muscles, they, by their strength, build your chest box to its optimum size. Even more important, they will keep it in this condition at all times so that your improved lungs are capable of utilizing the greater space to absorb a larger quantity of oxygen. In this way, your daily and nightly unconscious breathing act can become as formidable as is your conscious act.

Breathe exclusively through your nose at all times. Of course, under the stress of a great exertion, the body cells, mostly in the muscles, work very rapidly and consequently throw off more carbon dioxide. They produce it more rapidly than your lungs can get rid of it. The nerve center in your brain is alerted and makes you breathe faster and faster, and you begin to pant. You are no longer able to breathe in and out through your nose; your mouth automatically opens to compensate, and you begin inhaling and exhaling entirely through your mouth rather than imposing an unnecessary strain on your heart. It is perfectly natural to breathe with your mouth under stress and foolish to try to breathe solely through your nostrils.

If the nasal passages are completely blocked because of some obstruction, inspiration should then be practiced through the mouth and expiration through the nose. Under normal circumstances, oral or mouth breathing should be avoided, along with unnecessary holding of breath.

A basic rule to follow while exercising for coordinating movement with breathing, is to inhale as the arms move *away* from the body or sides, and to exhale as they return *toward* the sides or the starting position. In all waist-bending movements, exhale as you bend forward, and inhale as you raise your torso to the starting position.

The habit of deep breathing can be cultivated at odd moments during the day. When you are out walking, mentally count six paces, breathing deeply through your nose at the same time. Breathe out during the next six or eight paces. Give this method a thorough test and you will notice how quickly a feeling of warmth is induced, especially on a cold day. If you are breathing correctly, your waistline should expand as your diaphragm moves down; then the muscles in your back and sides should lift and expand the ribs; and finally, your chest should rise, completing one full breath. Once this becomes habitual, you will not need to make a special effort to breathe properly or deeply; it will have become a part of your nature.

Proper Posture
Is a Vital Necessity

Too much cannot be written about the health-giving qualities of proper posture. In my opinion, a large percentage of human ailments result directly from improper carriage of the body. The spine can be the seat of more bodily ills than any other section of the human frame.

One of the most basic requirements for a healthy and strong body throughout life is good posture. Therefore, emphasis on proper body position cannot be overdone.

Faulty posture over a long period of time produces deleterious effects on all of the functions of the body. Fatigue, headaches, backaches, and disturbances of the heart and the digestive and respiratory systems can be caused by this common fault. On the other hand, better health and mental and physical alertness are associated with proper posture.

You should make a habit of correct posture—in standing, walking, sitting, and lying. In all these body positions you should endeavor to be "tall." Hold your head up, neck back, chin in, chest up (but not out), back straight, shoulders relaxed and not thrown back, knees straight, and feet parallel and pointing forward with your weight resting on the outer edge of the feet. Try to maintain this standing position in a natural and relaxed manner. When sitting, and whenever it is necessary to lean forward (as in writing, etc.), lean forward from the hips without bending

14

at the waist. When lying down, stretch out fully without a
pillow, and avoid all bent or cramped positions.

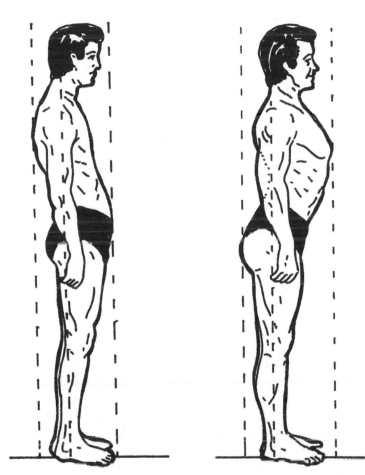

Fig. 1. Incorrect standing position commonly observed in
both men and women.

Fig. 2. Exaggerated standing
position which distorts both
spine and chest.

A good method of bringing your spine into the proper
position is to stretch your arms as high overhead as

possible. This naturally lifts the chest, and to some extent the head, so that the spine is pulled erect. Maintain this position for a moment, fixing the position of your back in your mind, then lower your arms. This can be performed at any time and in all of the above-mentioned body positions.

However, merely trying to maintain proper body position is scarcely sufficient to build the degree of strength that will hold your body up for long periods without any particular effort. Maintaining correct posture depends mainly on the normal coordination of the different muscles which support the body in an erect position.

Poor posture may be the result of flat feet, weak back muscles, a protruding abdomen, or any other muscular weakness of the body. These deformities are often correctable if a serious effort is made to overcome the weakness through intelligently applied exercise.

In short, the requirement for correct posture is a harmonious development of all the muscles of the body brought about by properly performed exercise designed to meet the individual's requirements.

During the many years I have spent in building better bodies, I have found that correct posture is one of the main requirements for good health. It is my candid opinion that poor posture is responsible for many organic troubles in the body. In case after case, I have proved conclusively that when poor posture is corrected many other ailments in the body are automatically eliminated. So watch your posture: sit straight, walk erect, and do not slouch over.

Proper carriage of the body

The importance of assuming a proper position at all times, whether sitting or standing, should be thoroughly understood. The proper carriage of the body for avoiding

and correcting round shoulders is shown in Fig. 3. This
position is one that can be especially recommended. The
shoulders should be back. The abdomen should not be
drawn in as is commonly recommended, but should be

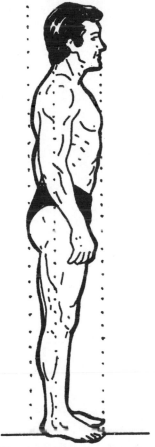

Fig. 3. Correct standing position, showing a natural and forcible
carriage of the body.

relaxed and perfectly free to move outward and inward as
the breath is inhaled and exhaled. There should be no
strain in any part. Correct position in both sitting and
standing is not only necessary to avoid round shoulders,

but also for the best general health. Study the position shown in Fig. 3 and try to maintain a proper position at all times.

Basic Foundation
Conditioning

Exercise to condition the body is a very important act in the life of every individual. The average person in search of health and strength is profoundly confused about trying to find and adopt an exercise program. There are many systems, and the claims made for some are so exaggerated and confusing that they leave the would-be pursuer bewildered.

One group of people believes that ordinary labor is enough to keep the body in good physical condition. If a limited amount of work or labor is performed energetically there may be some physical benefit, but the wrecked and shapeless bodies of millions of people stand out as incontestable evidence that work cannot replace systematic physical training.

There are many who think that games and sports can take the place of rational body conditioning. Athletic participation is fine for those individuals whose bodies are geared and trained to withstand the strenuous effort. Unfortunately, the average male or female is what I term a "weekend" athlete. After spending all week practically motionless behind a desk, they attempt to play a fast game of handball, tennis, or any other game on their days off in order to make up for a week of inactivity.

The same can be said for the "vacation" or "holiday" athletes. They spend fifty weeks of the year in a sedentary fashion, and try to balance the year's inactivity during two weeks of vacation. This is both foolish and dangerous. Permanent damage to the heart and other vital organs of the body can easily result from such overexertion. This type of radical performance is what gives exercise a bad name. There is nothing wrong with the activity; the incorrect application of it by the individual and his poor physical condition are at fault. If we are interested in the welfare of our bodies we must practice a program of conditioning exercises that will result in physical construction rather than physical destruction.

Many so-called instructors have the erroneous idea that calisthenic exercises are proper for conditioning the untrained. This approach is quite deceptive and may even prove harmful in some cases. The movements are too fast and out of rhythm with the respiratory tempo, and often leave the subject trembling and panting for breath. In the conditioning stage this type of exercise takes too long, employs far too many repetitions per exercise, and does not involve the proper muscular action. Calisthenics can be employed *after* the conditioning period is completed, but before then you must remember that the body is in an untoned condition, and is only accustomed to a few daily body movements. Movements of a too vigorous nature at the beginning will result in unnecessary discomfort.

The size and strength of a man offers no proof that he is internally sound. Therefore, preliminary training is a precautionary step in any conditioning program. The first step is to tone the internal organs and at the same time gradually accustom all the muscles to the varied movements of which they are capable without causing any stiffness or discomfort to appear.

This groundwork of conditioning is begun with a series of exercises that combine physical movements with concentrated respiration, producing a coordination of the internal and external muscular systems. In the beginning we are only concerned with performing the mildest of stimulative exercises, on the lowest scale of physical progression, as we are dealing with the most important organs to human life—the heart and the lungs. I have often heard the thorax or chest described as the zone of vitality. The health and the organic resistance of any individual depends upon the relation between his thorax and his whole body. A narrow chest is an indication that one's physiological entirety is weak. With an impaired chest condition the breathing function becomes shallow, and oxygen, the paramount element of life, is not sufficiently supplied to meet the bodily needs. The blood stream becomes impoverished and toxic due to the excessive amounts of carbon dioxide which are allowed to accumulate in the body. This deficient condition brings on fatigue, weakness, nervousness, etc.

Breathing must be efficient

The entire body depends upon the working efficiency of the respiratory system. After inhalation, the cells of the body receive a supply of oxygen to carry out their vital work through the medium of the blood stream. The exhalation of air out of the lungs, which rids the body of poisonous carbon dioxide, is equally important. How well the acts of inhaling and exhaling are carried out depends on the healthy functioning of the lungs and the condition of the muscles which mold the chest.

Externally, powerful muscles clothe the thoracic frame, serving partly in the movements of respiration and partly in the movements of the upper limbs. The most important muscle is the diaphragm, which completely closes the thoracic cavity, rising into it as a convex vault and separating it from the abdomen. It is the most active of the muscles which participate in the movements of respiration.

Before anyone can proceed safely with any form of activity or physical training, no matter how weak or strong the individual may be, he must perform the basic preliminary training exercises so that his body will be internally physically fit to withstand the increased demands which will be imposed on it when more vigorous exercises are practiced.

Progressive exercise is the only corrective agency which can permanently build a strong, healthy, beautiful body which can function with greater freedom and to the fullest of its natural capacity.

Nature works with constructive exercise, and the exercises illustrated are natural and scientifically adapted to develop the muscular system and vital organs. I want you to accept these exercises and practice them with confidence in the good they will do you.

Many of my readers may not be interested in all-around physical development; nevertheless, everyone should be interested in building up their vital sources to the best of their ability. In other words, every man, woman, and child should strive for body development, if only for health's sake.

Please do not become confused when I talk of the word "muscle." I do not mean, or intend, that your development shall be that of a super-strong man. The development of muscle is *always* within your control. By following the proper exercises, you can build muscle structure to the size and strength that best suits you, and *you can stop when you are satisfied.* On the other hand, if you wish to develop to greater proportions, that is your privilege and possibility. Only you can control this, and when the desired stage in development is reached, all you have to do is perform fewer repetitions of the exercise. Simply continue to exercise enough to keep fit and keep your body in its newly acquired, healthy state.

Dumbbells are prescribed for use with certain exercises, because a little weight supplies the resistance required to make the muscles function. Suit yourself as to the amount of weight you use, depending on your age and on your goals. A woman or a growing boy may use from one to three pounds in each hand. A man who seeks physical fitness without a display of muscle may use five- to ten-pound dumbbells. The middle-aged man should use no more than five-pound bells, unless he is very vigorous and *knows* he can easily handle more weight. The young man who is out for complete development will use dumbbells that provide him with a progressive range of resistance according to his increasing powers of muscular efficiency. In this case, it is best to own a pair of adjustable dumbbells or a barbell set that can be increased in jumps of a few pounds at a time. In this way, persons of both sexes and all ages can practice to their satisfaction according to the benefits in health, strength, and efficiency that they wish to attain.

Unfortunately, the average person has been taught to believe that using dumbbells or barbells is the wrong thing to do—a method too heavy for his particular need. In this he is decidedly wrong. Somehow it does not occur to him that either dumbbells or barbells can be made light enough for anyone despite his or her age or condition just as easily as they can be made heavy enough for the strongest.

The beauty of progressive weight resistance is that this method can be gauged and controlled to suit the body-building purpose of each individual. He can become fit to the point of personal satisfaction more rapidly by this than by any other method. Once he has arrived at the state desired, it is not necessary to go further into the advanced stages of training unless he wishes to do so.

Time is a very important factor which should never be overlooked. Progressive weight training requires only about one-fourth of the time calisthenics demand, and, instead of training morning and night, it is only necessary to train every other day.

There is no secret: simply determine to build your body the natural progressive way and you will not be disappointed. You will enjoy organic and muscular vigor when those who are victims of their own ignorance or prejudice are gone and forgotten.

Progress *gradually!* Do not seek to jump ahead at the beginning. A modern progressive course of organic strengthening exercises will surely build you to the stage when you can readily engage in the most vigorous activities and more than hold your own.

I wish to emphasize that the following exercises are only a method of preliminary body conditioning, and that the performer should not object to the light nature of the exercises. *Premature* exercise practice is detrimental to health, strength, and development.

Vitality-Building Exercises

Setting up an internal massage

Exercise 1. Lie on your back on the floor, with your body stretched out to its normal limit and your arms held by your sides. Before attempting the movement, breathe in quickly three or four times to prepare your lungs for the exercise.

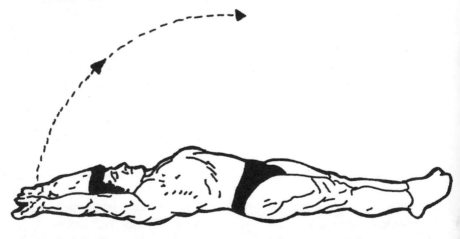

Conditioning Exercise 1

From this position, slowly raise your arms over your head, and continue without pause until the backs of your hands touch the floor behind your head. Keep breathing in from the moment your arms leave your sides until your hands touch the floor at the back of your head, when your lungs should be filled to their capacity.

Without stopping, begin to breathe out and at the same time allow your arms to travel back to their original position at the sides of your body. Exhalation should be complete as your arms reach the floor. Practice this movement six times in succession—but do it slowly throughout. Do not force your breathing or your physical action. Your arms must be kept straight throughout the exercise.

As your arms travel past your head and stretch behind it in the initial movement, you will feel a pressure in your diaphragm—the area of your stomach. This is caused by chest expansion in your lower rib box, which makes the relaxed abdominal muscles fall in and press upward, thereby lifting the lower portion of your lungs in a natural way to receive air and cooperate with the act of breathing in. You could not perform this movement as well standing, since you would require abdominal muscular contraction to do so, which an undeveloped body is incapable of. In the prone position you obtain benefit without exerting physical force, and at the same time you set up an internal massage with the action of your concealed muscles.

Stimulating the natural process of evacuation

Exercise 2. Remain in the same position as in movement No. 1, but wedge the back of your hands under the edge of your buttocks. Breathe in quickly three or four times as a preliminary stepping-up act. Keep your legs straight and rigid, and, without bending your knees, raise them towards your head.

Begin to breathe in as you raise your legs, and complete

the inhalation as your legs reach their limit of travel towards your head. If you are obese, your legs will barely travel past a line drawn at a right angle to your hips. If your weight is normal, they will go beyond that line. It is never necessary to go beyond the limit of 45° past the perpendicular to the hips. To touch your toes behind your head is to turn a natural movement into an acrobatic act, and this has no value.

After you have raised both legs fully, lower your legs slowly to the floor keeping in tempo with your breathing out.

Keep your legs straight throughout this exercise and do not try to force your legs to travel beyond the limit of your ability. Your body is an obstruction, and there is no purpose in pushing against a natural obstruction. As your muscles develop, all unnatural conditions will be naturally remedied.

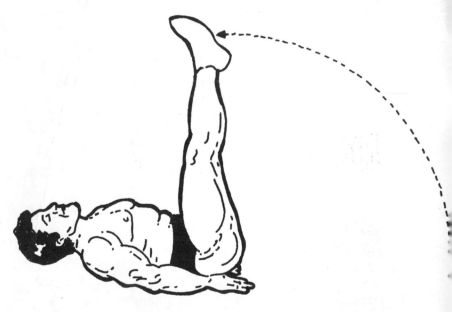

Conditioning Exercise 2

This movement develops the muscles below the line of your navel into your groin. Incidentally, these are the *weakest* muscles in your abdominal structure. Deterioration of these muscles causes prolapse of the abdomen, and leaves you an easy prey to rupture. With prolapse of your abdomen, your transverse colon—that very important tract of your intestinal system—loses its natural support and can sometimes drop to the floor of your pelvis, creating a dangerous condition by obstructing evacuation.

Practice this movement six times in succession, breathing in and out naturally, without forcing, throughout the entire exercise. This is the preparatory movement to condition the muscles of your abdomen safely and tone your intestinal system, stimulating the natural process of evacuation.

Note: If raising both legs proves too difficult at the start, raise your right leg and left leg alternately.

Limbering the life organs in your pelvic area

Exercise 3. Lie on one side for this movement. If you choose to start lying on your left side, then see that your right leg is placed on your left leg in the corresponding position. Your left arm should be placed a little in front of your body with the palm of your hand on the floor to

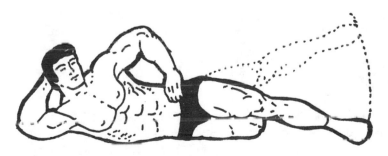

Conditioning Exercise 3

prevent your body from rolling as you perform the movement.

From this position, slowly begin to raise your right leg as high as possible, always in line with your left leg. Breathe in deeply, but naturally, as your leg is raised, and breathe out as your leg is lowered.

Practice this movement six times in succession, then reverse your position so that you lie on your right side and raise your left leg in the prescribed movement.

This exercise seems very simple, but you will be amazed at your limited ability to raise your leg to any appreciable extent. The fact is that your hip muscles are probably incapable of moving the thighbone in the hip socket. Deterioration of muscular mechanics and energy in this region creates a pronounced deficiency in the important life organs encased within your pelvic area, and this has a detrimental influence upon your whole body. People stiffen in the hips readily, which is why it is said that people begin to age first in the legs.

To tone your sacral and lumbar regions: The small of your back

Exercise 4. Stand with your feet spaced about 18 inches apart, and your hands cupped on the hips. Hold your chin up, and start off by taking three or four quick breaths.

From this position, bend sideways *without swaying your hips*—first to the left side, then to the right side, and then bend forward with your back straight, no further than at a right angle to your body.

Perform these three movements in a slow, rhythmic, 1–2–3 order. The breathing act cannot be applied to the three movements in this exercise, but you should breathe in and out as naturally and slowly as you can while you perform these movements successively.

Practice this movement six times, that is, six times in each direction, making a total of 18 movements.

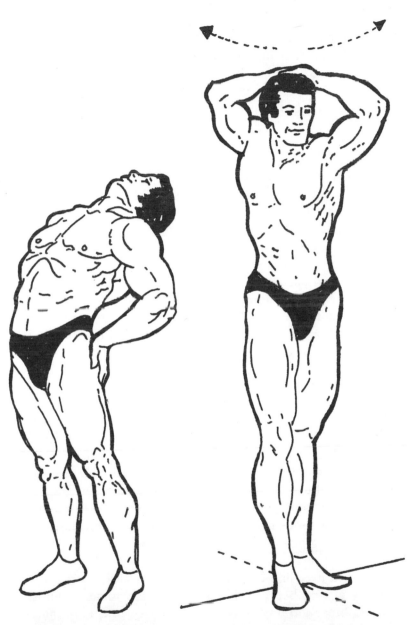

Conditioning Exercise 4   Conditioning Exercise 5

The object of this exercise is to further loosen up your hips, and loosen the vertebral section in the small of your back; termed the sacral and lumbar area. Fatigue toxin makes its deepest inroads here, which you experience as back aches and pains, hip stiffness, and a weariness that creates the desire to drop into a chair and ease your back, or "take the weight off your feet."

Vitality-building exercises for the waist and spinal column

In these movements the hips and the legs should remain in their original position facing forwards and should not move with the trunk.

Exercise 5. Stand erect with your hands clasped behind your head. Then turn your whole trunk to the right, moving from your hips up. Twist back past the face-forward position and turn your trunk fully to the left. Repeat four to six times in each direction.

Exercise 6. Stand erect with your hands clasped behind your head. Then bend your whole trunk to the right from your hips. Swing back past the upright position and bend it fully to the left. Repeat four to six times in both directions.

Exercise 7. Stand erect with your hands on the hips or at your sides. Then, without moving your legs or the lower part of the body below the hips, bend forward as far as possible. Next bring the body back past the upright position and carry it backwards as far as possible. Repeat four to six times. Breathe out slowly and completely when bending forward and at the same time try to pull in your abdomen without straining. Inhale on the returning motion, relaxing your abdomen at the same time.

Note. You may find it difficult to follow these instructions strictly at first because of stiffness in the spine, shoulder joints, hips and knees, or weakness in the abdominal muscles. But no matter how little progress you make at first, steadily persist in your efforts to overcome these conditions. You will be amply rewarded.

These exercises aim at improving your muscle tone, posture and flexibility.

In all exercises where breathing is not mentioned breathe naturally and normally, and try not to hold your breath.

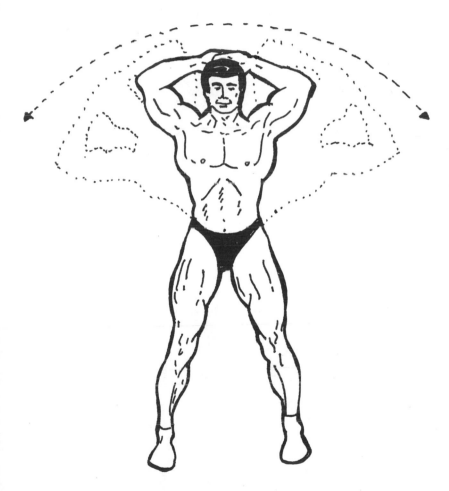

Conditioning Exercise 6

Exercise 8. Stand erect. Place the right palm over the right buttock and the left palm over the left buttock, as illustrated. Now slowly tense the buttock muscles, and at the same time draw them together as tightly as possible. Hold them tight for a moment and slowly release the tension. Repeat this movement at least three or four times. Rest and do it again.

Note: Try to sense how the buttocks become firm in

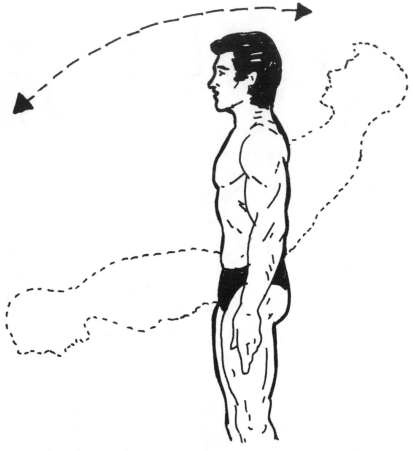

Conditioning Exercise 7

tension, against the palms, and how they soften as they are being relaxed. Keep in mind that the release of muscles should be as much under control as their contraction.

Exercise 9. Practically all exercise movements should be co-ordinated with buttock control. The tension and release

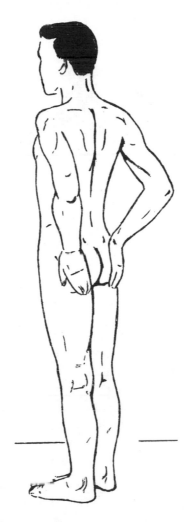

Conditioning Exercise 8

control of the buttock muscles will aid in tightening their outline and reducing the unsightly flabby mass.

Acquire the habit of tightening the buttocks while walking, sitting, and when reaching for something overhead.

The buttock muscles connect the legs with the upper part of the body and play a most important part in moving the trunk while walking and climbing stairs. Therefore their condition and development will help to prevent back problems.

Exercise 10. Stand erect with your hands clasped behind your head. Without moving any part of your body below the hips, rotate your trunk on your hips, beginning the rotation to the left and making as wide a circle of movement as possible. Continue the rotation for a short period and then reverse the direction, so that the rotation begins to the right. Continue for a short period in this direction.

Exercise 11. Stand erect with your hands clasped behind your head. Then, without moving your trunk and without bending your legs in any direction, move your hips out to the right to their fullest extent. Bring them back past the normal position, and move them out to the left to the fullest extent. Repeat four to six times.

Exercise 12. Stand erect with your hands clasped behind your head. Then, without moving the upper part of your body or your legs, rotate your hips, beginning the rotation to the right and making as big a circle of movement with them as possible. After a short period of rotating in this direction, begin a new rotation to the left and continue the circle of movement in that direction for a short period.

Vitality-building exercises for activating the hip joints

Exercise 13. Stand erect with your arms dropped to a natural position at your sides and your legs slightly apart.

Then lift your right leg from the ground without bending it in any way or carrying it either forwards or backwards. Let it be drawn up by the hip joint to the furthest capacity of the joint. From the farthest upward point, lower the leg to the fullest extent possible without allowing the foot to touch the ground. The leg is not lifted outwards in any

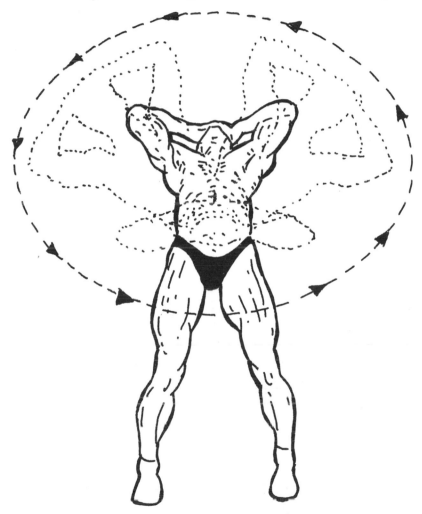

Conditioning Exercise 10

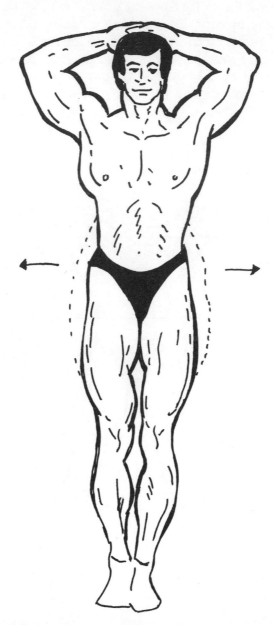

Conditioning Exercise 11

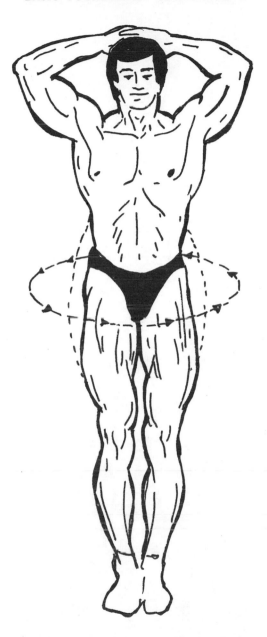

Conditioning Exercise 12

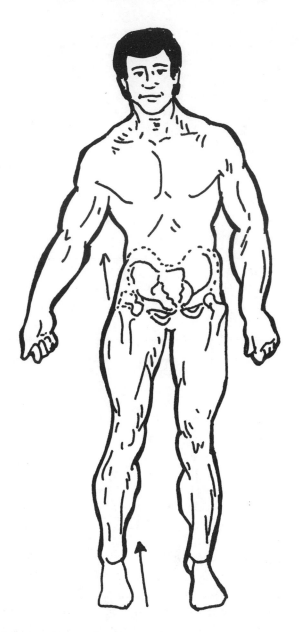

Conditioning Exercises 13 and 14

way, but is merely drawn up parallel with the other leg, and the whole of the movement is impelled by the hip joint.

Exercise 14. Repeat exactly as for exercise 13, using the left leg instead of the right for the movement. Repeat four to six times.

Exercise 15. Stand erect with your hands clasped behind your head and your feet together. Then relax the knee joint of your left leg, bending your leg at the knee, so that your left hip is carried downwards to the lowest possible point, while your right leg remains unbent and your right hip joint bears the weight of your body. Then transfer the weight of your body to your left hip joint, allowing your right knee joint to relax and bend and your right hip joint to sag down as far as possible.

This movement is actually a shifting of body weight from one hip to the other. The movement should be done on the balls of the feet without lifting either foot from the ground. Jerking of any kind is to be avoided. Repeat four to six times.

Vitality-building exercises for the legs

Exercise 16. Stand erect with your arms hanging naturally at your sides and your feet together. Gradually bend your knees with the weight of your body slowly going down, but without allowing your trunk to bend forward. Continue the lowering movement until you have sunk into a sitting position on your heels. During this movement your heels will spontaneously lift from the ground, so that by the time you have reached a sitting position you will be on your toes. From this sitting position rise slowly to your original standing position, keeping your trunk erect.

This movement requires care that your body does not drop to the sitting position. Let the muscles of your legs perform the entire movement slowly and completely. Repeat four to six times.

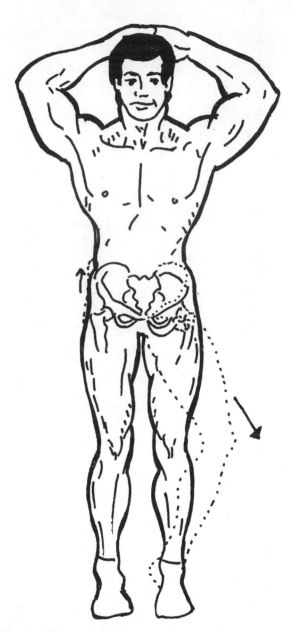

Conditioning Exercise 15

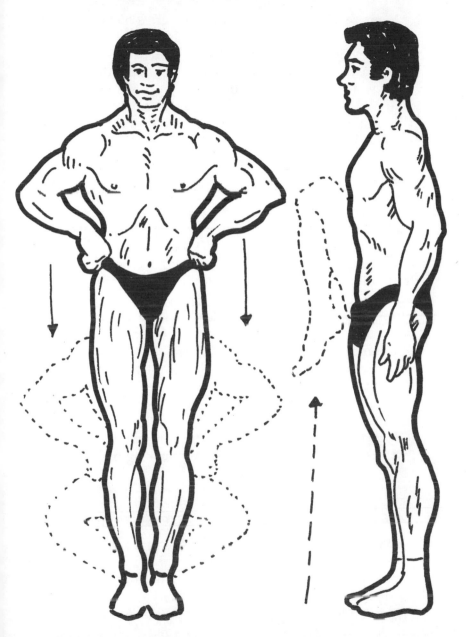

Conditioning Exercise 16   Conditioning Exercise 17

Exercise 17. Stand erect with your arms hanging naturally at your sides. Then bring your legs up alternately in an exaggeration of the movement used to climb stairs, carrying your legs up to the highest point possible. In this movement, your knees should come up enough to strike your chest with ease. The leg joints are not fully freed until you can do this without bending your body forward. Repeat four to six times.

Exercise 18. Stand erect and, rising on your toes, spring a short pace to the left on your left foot, and then back again onto your right foot, with your right foot placed at the distance of a short pace to the right. After springing from side to side in this manner for a while, change the movement to a forward and backward springing so that you are actually springing a short pace forward and backward from foot to foot. After a while reverse the position of your feet in the forward and backward springing so that whichever foot carried the forward spring now carries the backward one, and vice versa.

The best results from this movement can be obtained by varying the directions and changing feet frequently. Keep in mind not to rush through the movements.

In this movement it is particularly important to stop at the first hint of a feeling of tiredness. On the other hand, if it does not seem to make a sufficient call on your limbs at first, you may counterbalance this by making the stride of your spring wider.

Vitality-building exercises for shoulder joints and muscles

Exercise 19. Stand erect with your arms fully extended above your head. From this position, reach up with your arms until your shoulder joints are lifted to their fullest possible extent, without lifting your heels from the ground or moving the lower part of your body in any way. Then, still keeping your arms up, bring your shoulder joints

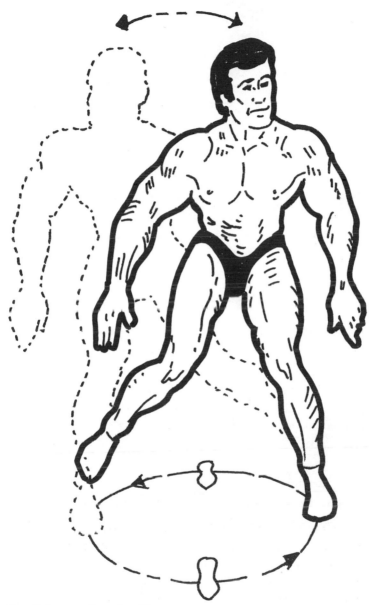

Conditioning Exercise 18

down until they are lowered to their fullest possible extent. Repeat four to six times.

Exercise 20. Stand erect with your arms extended forward at the height of your shoulders. Then, without moving your body, reach forward with your arms until your shoulder joints are moved forward to their fullest extent. Then, without bringing in your arms, draw your shoulder joints back until they are pulled back to their fullest extent. Repeat four to six times.

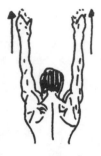

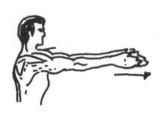

Conditioning Exercise 19   Conditioning Exercise 20

Exercise 21. Stand erect with your arms fully extended sideways at the height of your shoulders. Then, without moving your body, reach out with your hands so that your shoulder joints are thrust outward to their fullest possible extent. Next, without bringing in your arms, draw your

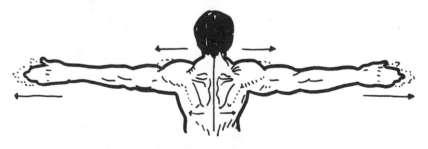

Conditioning Exercise 21

shoulder joints in until they are fully pulled in. Repeat four to six times.

Exercise 22. Stand erect with your arms hanging naturally at your sides. Without moving any other part of your body, lift your shoulder joints to the highest extent possible. With your arms still hanging at your sides, carry your shoulder joints down from the highest to the lowest point possible. Repeat four to six times.

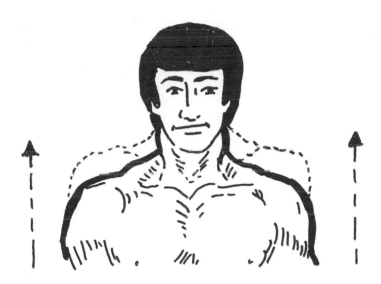

Conditioning Exercise 22

Exercise 23. Stand erect with your arms hanging naturally at your sides. Without moving your body, rotate your shoulder joints forward, making as large a circle of movement as possible, without allowing your arms to move in any way except as they are carried by the shoulder joints. Repeat a number of times and then reverse the rotation so that it moves backwards. Repeat a number of times in that direction.

Exercise 24. Stand erect with your arms resting natu-

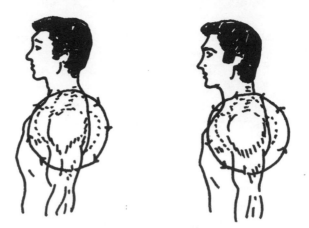

Conditioning Exercise 23

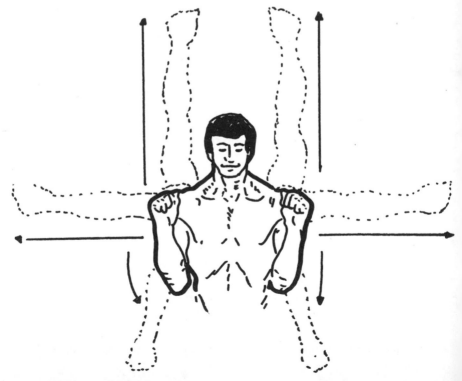

Conditioning Exercise 24

rally at your sides. Bring them up to your chest and stretch them upward; bring them back to your chest and stretch them out to the sides; back to your chest and out to the front; back to your chest and down at the sides; back to your chest and as far and as high as possible backward without disturbing the poise of your body. Repeat a number of times and gradually work up to 18 repetitions.

Exercise 25. Stand erect with your arms extended outwards at shoulder level. Then bring your arms in together across your chest, one passing immediately above the other. Swing them out to the fully extended position and bring them in again, but with the arm that passed above the other on the previous swing now passing below. Repeat four to six times with the arms alternately passing above and below each other.

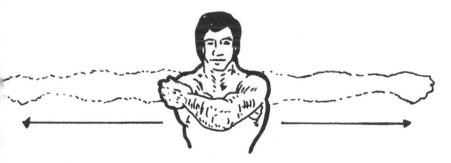

Conditioning Exercise 25

Important points to remember: Those who have not previously done any exercises of this type must first gradually tone the muscular condition of their body and organs. Those who have had previous experience will have a slight advantage at first over the novice, but it is still wise for them to be careful. Only those who take time and patience to build a substantial foundation during the first few weeks will achieve success.

Practice the first four exercises for at least seven days.

Then add another four to six exercises and practice them for two weeks; gradually complete the entire 25 movements in this progression. Do some in the morning and a few in the evening. Keep with the first four exercises as the basis of this precautionary system of training. It is best to proceed slowly and safely. Be sure to understand each exercise and perfect your performance before trying the next one. The wrong application makes the effort worthless.

Important General Pointers to Observe

There are over five hundred muscles in the human body. For development and bodybuilding purposes they are classified in groups, such as chest, abdominal, back, neck, leg, and arm muscles.

You will find that each chapter or section is a course in itself, devoted to building a particular area of the body. Each type of exercise is also divided up into three or four groups of elementary, medium, and advanced movements.

After several weeks of faithfully practicing and mastering the precautionary or conditioning exercises outlined, you will be prepared to start the progressive, gradated movements.

It is important that you study the illustrations and instructions carefully. The illustrations show the exercises being perfectly performed. Don't get discouraged if you find it difficult to duplicate them. Consistent practice in front of a mirror is of considerable help in eliminating your faults by comparing your performance with the illustrations.

Select two or three exercises which involve different sections of the body from each of the "A" groups. Practice eight to ten exercises each day and vary them over a period of several weeks until you have perfected your performance in all of them. The same method should be followed for the "B" group, "C" group, etc.

In the beginning it is wise to rest one day per week. As you ascend the scale of physical progression and lift heavier weight per exercise it is best to rest twice a week. After exercising steadily for three months it is best to "lay off" for a week, giving your body a chance to rest and rebuild with renewed enthusiasm and determination.

Never exercise to the point of exhaustion; do not allow enthusiasm and overambition to carry you beyond the bounds of practical requirement and common sense.

You may have lowered pep and energy on certain days. Don't confuse this lack of pep with laziness. If you are unable to perform an exercise the prescribed number of times, let your condition be your guide and perform the movement fewer times.

Keep a record of the exercises you perform, how many times you repeat them, and how much weight you are using. This will help you to maintain an accurate schedule and will give you a clear idea of the gains you make. Remember, physical fitness or physical development can be improved by gradually increasing the amount of work performed, but you must progress in easy stages. Overdoing an exercise or training program will retard progress. You should never attempt to lift a heavy weight until you have gradually trained and conditioned yourself to do so.

Before beginning the actual training programs, you would be wise to devote some time to perfecting the exercise positions and determining the right amount of weight to use for each exercise.

There are two ways of holding a dumbbell or barbell. The undergrip (palms up) allows the bell to rest in the palm of your hand as you raise the bell. In the overgrip (palms down), you hold the bar with your knuckles above the bar and your thumbs below. The barbell is usually held with the hands a shoulder width apart.

It is almost impossible to advise you on the correct amount of weight to use for each exercise. No two persons are alike; age, weight, condition, and occupation differ.

You must use your own judgment, starting out with poundages per exercise well within your limits. From this point, you will learn to select the amount of weight which you can handle correctly for the scheduled number of repetitions and still complete your training session without feeling fatigued—just comfortably tired.

After you have attained a considerable degree of improvement, you can step up your schedule by repeating an exercise or entire routine over again. This is termed a set, and you can do two or three sets of the same routine.

Exercise in a well-ventilated room, free of drafts. If the room is too cold for muscular warmth, wear light, loose, porous training clothes, as they allow greater air circulation.

You may exercise at any time provided it does not interfere with your regular meals or sleeping hours. You should allow at least one or two hours to elapse after eating before indulging in a training session.

The length of your workout will depend on your physical condition and on how hard you train. At the most, a short rest of one minute between exercises should suffice. Make sure your muscles are kept warm during rest periods. A sweat shirt or exercise suit is perfect for this. Do not rush through your exercises. Remember to make your workout consistent for best results.

Take a warm and cool shower after you complete your exercise session, followed by a brisk toweling. This will stimulate surface circulation and have a beneficial effect on your skin.

If there is any part of your body that appears to lack balance, ignore it until you have completed your entire training program, to give the underdeveloped part a chance to respond. If it fails to respond satisfactorily to your complete program, you can begin to consider exercise specialization to bring the underdeveloped muscles up to par and provide perfect symmetry to your body.

Turn to "Know Your Muscles." Study the anatomical

charts and then look up the corresponding exercises and activities for specific parts of the body. If you find that one part has not developed satisfactorily you should specialize on that part.

The following method of specialization has helped many, and it may give you an idea of how to proceed in this direction. It is a 30-day program divided into two-week parts. Select four to six exercises for the muscles you wish to improve and practice them for two weeks. Practice each exercise 12 times, performing the first four repetitions with whatever weight you select to begin with. Increase the weight by five pounds for the next four counts, and increase the weight by another five pounds for the last four counts.

During the second two-week training period you should increase the step up per exercise and use more weight. Perform the first three repetitions with whatever weight you select to begin with. For the second, third, and fourth sets increase the weight by 7½ pounds for each set.

The weight increases given are average ones. The increases can be greater if you are specializing on your leg or back muscles, but you will have to judge this for yourself. In some cases, such as exercises for the abdomen and neck, where less weight is used than for the arms, chest, back, or legs, the increases should be less. This is also a matter for you to determine according to your own ability. Do not strain, but go all out and make your muscles really work.

Treasure Your Chest

The most vital organs of life are contained in the chest. A well-developed chest means greater health and beauty for you.

How's your chest development? Is it deep, full and high? Is it several inches larger than your waistline? These are good questions because your chest development is a very good indication of your vitality and physical status.

Your chest is not merely a cage of bones. It is a marvelous, integral part of the human anatomy. The heart and lungs are housed within the chest walls. The external muscles provide adequate protection against injury to these organs, as well as giving the chest that beautiful appearance. Coordinately, the inner and outer mechanisms are constantly carrying out the vital processes of life. Therefore, everyone should strive to possess a well-developed chest.

Individuals whose chests are small, flat, and depressed cannot be robust and healthy. The breathing function becomes shallow with an impaired chest condition. Not enough oxygen is supplied to meet the bodily needs. The blood stream becomes impoverished and toxic due to the excess of carbon dioxide which is allowed to accumulate in the body. So, when the supply of oxygen diminishes, the vitality and health of the body is also diminished.

This brings us to the very important and serious matter of why chest development is indispensable to bodily health and strength.

Life is movement. If the activity of any part of the body falls below par, it will grow less capable of performing its function. The chest is no exception to this law. It will become depressed and contracted; the muscles will become weak, shortened and rigid; the tissue and air cells of the lungs will gradually atrophy from want of expansion and recoil; and the evil effects of shallow breathing will become evident. Without ample air, every cell and vital function will become sluggish and weak.

To build and maintain a healthy chest, you must make it work. To accomplish this, it is best to resort to rational exercise. Proper exercise will extend and strengthen the muscles of the chest in every way. With an increase in chest capacity, the heart and lungs will not be cramped, they will be able to carry out their work naturally, and they will respond more effectively and promptly to the demands placed upon them.

Many health enthusiasts rely upon voluntary breathing exercises while the body is held stationary to develop the chest. While breathing capacity is increased somewhat by this forced procedure, it does nothing to improve the chest permanently. Deep breathing taken simultaneously with muscular exercise creates a demand for oxygen, and at the same time develops the muscles which control the act of inhaling and exhaling.

You may not be interested in acquiring the large chest muscles of the athlete, but everyone should be interested in building normal chest development for health's sake. Your chest should be at least eight inches larger than your waist measurement. The super-developed bodybuilder often attains a difference of 12 inches, and sometimes more. However, this gain is largely from the increased development of the *latissimus* muscles which form the slab of the back and branch out sidewise from the chest, giving the upper body a V-shaped appearance. The average man should seek to build his chest until there is an eight-inch difference in circumference between his chest and waist.

Then he can truly say he is in perfect condition, but not before.

Since the chest contains the most vital organs of life—the heart and lungs—we will have to delve somewhat into its anatomy (structure) and physiology (function) to understand its kinetics or mechanics properly.

The thorax, as a whole, begins at the throat and extends downward to where the abdomen begins. It is composed of twelve pairs of ribs that appear to have a barrel shape.

Structurally, the walls of the chest are formed by a vertebral column (12 *dorsal* or *thoracic* vertebrae) in back, the breastbone or *sternum* in front, the ribs with their *intercostal* muscles around the sides, and the membranous and muscular diaphragm which divides the thorax from the abdomen below. The heads of the ribs form joints with the dorsal vertebrae, and the front ends of the ribs are connected to the sternum by the flexible costal cartilages. The backbone, sternum, and ribs form an elastic framework with movable sides. Thus the chest gives protection to the contained organs and assists largely in the process of respiration.

In addition to giving protection to the organs of respiration and circulation, the ribs give support to the bones of the shoulder girdle and upper extremities, and serve as an attachment for the chest and abdominal muscles.

The ribs are not positioned horizontally, but incline downwards from the backbone, and when they are raised and depressed during inspiration and expiration, the capacity of the chest is alternately increased and decreased.

The internal and external intercostal muscles assist in this coordinated muscular act by which the cavity of the chest is widened and deepened. There are eleven intercostal muscles on each side of the inner chest, occupying the spaces between the ribs and connecting the adjacent ribs throughout their length. The external intercostal muscles raise the ribs, widening the cavity of the chest and assisting inspiration. The internal intercostal muscles depress the ribs, making the chest narrower and assisting expiration.

Now let us go back and see how we can increase the chest size by a natural process. In order to do this, we must coordinate our exercises with the natural construction of the chest. To permanently increase the chest, the muscles that surround the chest must be exercised in such a manner that they not only spread the rib cage, but also accumulate muscular tissue to such a degree that they retain this growth. Exercises that simply spread or expand the chest, as in the case of all free movements, do not mean a thing. They undoubtedly cause a greater initial expansion, but this means nothing, since the heart and lungs do not acquire a larger permanent space for their functions. The most important muscles of the chest are the *pectorals* and the *serratus magnus* and as these muscles grow, the cartilages of the ribs become longer, thicker, and more secure in their attachment. As this process takes place, the chest becomes deeper, squarer, and higher. The muscular coat is heavier and more protective. These muscles are the real agents of chest growth, and since we have made ourselves fully familiar with rib construction and attachment to the extent that we know the course nature takes in promoting chest growth, we will pass on and study the whys and wherefores of these muscular agents, so that every chest builder can overcome all of his chest difficulties.

I used to read anatomy books, but I was completely swamped by the long technical names that are incomprehensible to the layman. Maybe this is the reason I take time, and perhaps more than necessary care, to explain it all to you in an understandable way, free of all technical phrases. A simple analysis will enable you to visualize where these muscles originate and become inserted, and you will then be able to realize how they operate.

The pectorals, or breastplate muscles, have a dual

function. They lift up the chest and contract it. In fact, they are so powerful in their contractile action that they are known as the crushing muscles of the body. While they are a great aid in all crushing movements of the arms, they are equally effective in resisting a crushing pressure. Many muscle builders take great pride in their pectoralis muscles, and develop them to extremes. When these particular athletes stand relaxed, their shoulders are pulled forward. While this does not have a detrimental effect on their chests because the other chest muscles are well developed, they are unsightly. Balanced development of all muscles enhances the beauty of the body and provides for balanced power.

The pectoralis muscles are also efficient in lifting the chest. The uplift action is known as the clavicular chest lift, since the pectorales are divided into two sections; the upper section is attached to the clavicle (or the collar bone) and the sternum (or breastbone). Therefore, your chest automatically lifts when you throw your shoulders back. This movement is familiar to the average person, since we lift our chests far more frequently than we expand them.

The serratus magnus muscles work to expand the chest. As we throw our shoulders back, breathe deeply, and push out the chest, the serratus magnus muscles lift and pull outward, causing the squareness to the chest so evident in strong, robust people. These muscles widen the lower section of the chest and give width to the diaphragm. This section, sometimes spoken of as the thoracic arch or chest bridge, is indicated by the bony curve over the stomach where the chest ends, and is probably the most important section of the chest. It is a sensitive part of our physical makeup. A punch there may knock out an undeveloped man quickly and painfully. Back in the early 1900s Heavyweight Boxing Champion Bob Fitzsimmons showed the boxing profession a new knockout route with this punch, and from then on boxers called it the solar plexus blow.

We all know that if the muscles are not developed within the thoracic arch the stomach will be left wide open to danger. Lack of muscular protection allows stomach distension, hernia, and prolapse. When a person has acquired diaphragm breathing depth he is capable of exercising his lung spaces completely. Such a person will be full of vital energy, vigorously strong, and physically efficient.

Before anyone can reach this stage of efficiency, he must have qualified through the other stages. To understand this, you must remember that there are four stages of breathing development. They are the clavicle stage, which takes place in the upper chest spaces; the intercostal stage, which takes place in the middle chest spaces; and the diaphragm stage, which takes place in the lower chest. The fourth stage is called the thoracic, and is really a combination of the first three stages, since the word thoracic refers to the entire chest scheme.

Normally, the average person rarely employs much more than the clavicle stage. A person who is more than ordinarily robust will employ more of the intercostal stage, but no one ever reaches the diaphragm stage except the chest-trained bodybuilder. The average deep breather never reaches diaphragm depth, since he lacks the muscular cooperation necessary for this.

Every man I have ever known who was a vital physical success had a finely proportioned chest. On the other hand, the flat or sunken chest is an unmistakable picture of low vitality and lack of resistance. You should strive to overcome any deficiencies in this area not only for the sake of physical comeliness and symmetry, but also because of its relation to the energy and stamina of the entire body and to the question of sustained health and life.

The real value of chest development lies in building the muscles of the chest, so that the chest is not only enlarged during exercise, but greater power is also permanently built into the muscles and they become capable of holding the increased depth, width, and uplift without any conscious effort on the part of the individual. The muscles are there for this purpose. Due to personal neglect on the part of the average individual, the muscles lose much of their natural strength, allowing the chest to sink and often resulting in a flat-chested condition. The chest walls become muscularly deficient more readily than does the breast of the chest, mainly because we employ the pectorals far more in daily movement than we do the serratus magnus muscles. Deficiency of the latter muscles is not so evident to the eye as is a flat chest, but it is there just the same.

Many slim people display what looks like a distended stomach; it really is not. The distention is caused by lack of width in the thoracic arch, which does not provide sufficient natural space for the stomach and forces it out. By simply widening the diaphragm with corrective exercise that strengthens the serratus magnus muscles, which in turn widens the thoractic arch and maintains it, this condition will be corrected.

To complete our kinetic analysis of chest building, we must consider the muscles of the back.

We have two *latissimi dorsi* and two *trapezius* muscles on our backs. The first named mean "broadest back muscles," and form the bulk of the back. Originating from the spine, they taper into a powerful tendon which is strongly fastened to the upper arm. These muscles are highly interesting to all weight lifters.

The trapezius is a peculiarly shaped muscle. It arises from the spine in a long taper, then triangles out to fasten onto the shoulder blade. From this connection it runs back up the neck and finally becomes attached to the base of the skull.

The powerful contraction of these two back muscles shortens the back, and this shortness is what deepens the chest, and squares and spreads the shoulders. For these reasons the back muscles must always be considered in molding a mighty chest.

Chest Exercise Without Apparatus

Group A

Practice the following exercises at least two hours after eating. See that your room is properly ventilated and that the air circulates freely. Watch your posture. Do not slouch over when exercising, or at any time.

Exercise 1. Stand erect with your arms held by your sides. Begin to breathe slowly, raising your arms rigidly up and over your head. While you are raising your arms, lift one leg as high as possible, bending it at the knee. Exhaling, return to original position. Alternate legs, and remember to move your legs in unison with your arms.

Exercise 2. Stand erect. Hook the middle finger of one hand with that of the other on a level with your waist and try to pull them apart. Still pulling, raise both arms to a position high over and above your head without straining.

Exercise 3. Stand erect. With your hands placed around an imaginary rope just above your head, pull downward, tensing your chest muscles. Keep your hands close together and pull down to your knees, keeping your body upright.

Exercise 4. Lie flat on your back with your body stretched out and your arms held by your sides. Slowly raise your arms rigidly, inhaling slowly, until the backs of your hands touch the floor behind your head. Slowly return your arms to their original position, breathing out.

Exercise 5. Stand erect with your arms held straight in front of you on a level with your shoulders. Breathe in deeply. Hold chest as high as possible. Cross your arms rigidly over your chest. Breathe out as your arms uncross and return to starting position. Alternate arms in crossing each other.

Exercise 6. While in a seated position, bend your arms and put your hands on your shoulders. Raise your arms overhead with the palms of your hands facing the ceiling, reaching as high as possible while breathing in. Return to your starting position while exhaling. While you are in this seated position, you should also grasp the seat with both hands and raise your body slightly, going up and down several times.

Exercise 7. Lie on the floor, facing down, and support your body on your hands and toes. Keep your entire body perfectly rigid. Lower it slowly, bending your arms until your chest touches the floor. Raise the body to starting position. If you cannot perform this exercise nine times at the start, simply do it until you are tired, and do not strain.

Each of these exercises should be performed at least nine times. Increase the number by one on every third practice night until 18 movements are performed. Those individuals who cannot reach the minimum repetitions should only perform the exercises until they are tired, and should not strain. It is very important that all the movements be in unison with breathing. Inhale slowly and deeply when exerting yourself and exhale fully when relaxing. Always breathe through your nose.

Chest Exercises With Apparatus

Group B

Exercise 1. Stand with your feet spaced apart, with the dumbbells between them. Bend over with your knees slightly bent and breathe out. While breathing in, swing the bells overhead, and simultaneously lunge forward into the position shown in the second drawing. From this overhead position, swing the bells down and far back between your legs, breathing out and at the same time bringing the forward leg back to its original position. Alternate legs in lunging forward. Your arms should swing freely and be kept in line with your shoulders throughout. You may bend your arms and knees a bit while in motion. Make sure to inhale completely on the upward swing, and exhale fully on the downward swing.

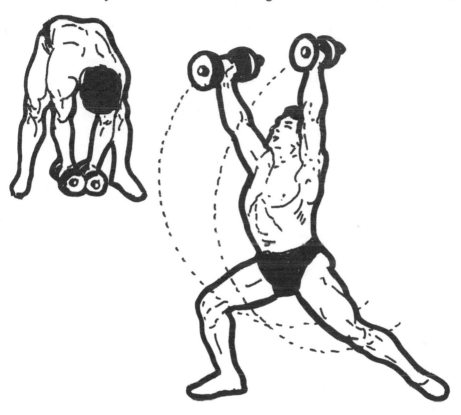

Chest Exercise B1

Repeat nine times. Add one repetition at every third practice session until you can perform 18 correctly, and then add five pounds to each bell and start over with nine repetitions.

This is a great warm-up exercise which can be used throughout the exercise program. A splendid all-around movement, it is especially good for the erector-spine muscles and the small of the back.

Exercise 2. Lie on your back with dumbbells held overhead at arm's length. Inhale fully and then slowly exhale, bringing the dumbbells over your head and keeping your arms straight until they rest at your sides. Inhale slowly and return to the starting position. You must breathe in and out fully, in unison with the arm movements, and keep your arms straight throughout the exercise.

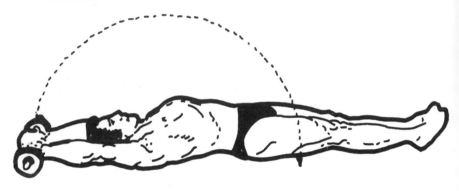

Chest Exercise B2

Repeat six times. Add one repetition at every third practice session until you can perform 14 counts, and then add 2½ pounds to each dumbbell and start over with six repetitions.

This exercise is excellent for the chest and shoulder muscles and for deepening the chest.

Exercise 3. Assume the position shown in the illustration, using a low stool. Breathing in slowly, lower your arms sideways until the dumbbells touch the floor. Breathe out slowly as your arms return to the overhead position. Hold your chest high and do not allow your legs to sag. Keep your arms straight throughout the exercise.

Practice six times. Add one repetition at every third

practice session until 18 counts are made, and then add 2½ pounds to each dumbbell and start over from the count of six.

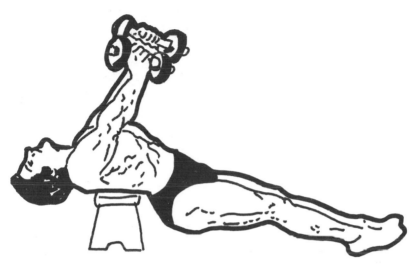

Chest Exercise B3

This exercise is excellent for the chest and shoulder muscles and for broadening the chest.

Exercise 4. Stand erect with your feet spaced comfortably apart, and your arms at your sides. Breathe in, crossing your rigid arms over your chest as far as possible without deflating your chest. Breathe out as your arms uncross to the original position. Keep your chest high, head well back, and arms straight. Breathe fully and deeply. Fifteen pounds is the maximum weight allowed with this exercise.

Repeat nine times. Add one repetition at every third practice session until 18 counts are reached, and then add 2½ pounds to each bell and start over with the original count of nine. This exercise aids *pectorale* development.

Exercise 5. Stand erect with your feet spaced comfortably apart and your arms held out straight in front and

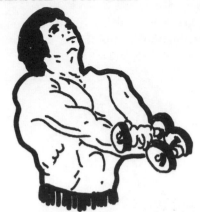

Chest Exercise B4

level with your shoulders. Breathe in slowly, bringing your arms outward and backwards as shown in the illustration. Breathe out slowly and fully as your arms return to their original position. Keep your arms straight throughout the exercise. It is not necessary to use more than 15 to 20 pounds with this exercise to receive maximum benefits.

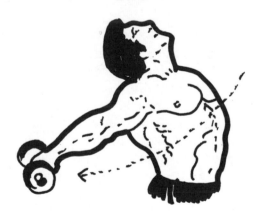

Chest Exercise B5

Repeat six times. Add one repetition at every third practice session until 14 counts are made, and then add 2½ pounds to each bell and start over from the original count of six.

This exercise is excellent for the chest muscles and for widening the rib box.

Exercise 6. Assume a sitting position with the dumbbells, as shown in the illustration. From this position, inhale and slowly raise the dumbbells to arm's length overhead. Breathe out as you lower the bells to your shoulders. Keep your back straight, and extend your arms upward fully. Do not let your heels leave the floor, and look up as you raise the bells.

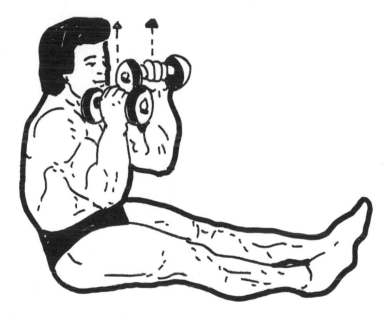

Chest Exercise B6

Repeat six times. Add one repetition at every third practice session until 12 counts are made, then add five pounds to each bell and start over from the original count of six.

This exercise is excellent for the back, chest, arms, and shoulders.

Exercise 7. Stand perfectly erect with your heels together and your arms by your sides, holding the dumbbells with the palms of your hands facing downwards. Slowly raise your arms forward and upward until they reach an overhead position, breathing in all the way. Exhale slowly as you return to the starting position. Keep your arms straight throughout and maintain an erect position.

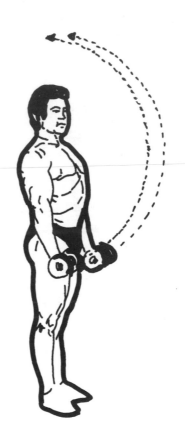

Chest Exercise B7

Repeat nine times and gradually work up to 18 repetitions, then add 2½ pounds to each bell and start over with the original count of nine.

The young man who wishes to obtain a more pronounced development of his chest and lungs can supplement his group B exercises with such sports as wrestling, swimming, handball, tennis, and running. An excellent method would be to continue the practice of dumbbell and barbell exercises, using weight resistance in graduated amounts, along with cable or chest-pull exercisers. The dipping movements outlined in "You, Too, Can Build Strong Arms" are excellent shoulder and chest builders.

Don't walk around with your chest forced out. You will not progress any faster. Try to maintain a correct body posture at all times—chest well forward, shoulders back, chin in and down, breathing deeply and fully without straining. When you exercise intelligently and consistently, you will get "chesty" naturally and with greatly improved health and strength.

Trim Your Waistline

The abdominal or waist region of the body has often been referred to as the center of health by numerous health and physical culture authorities, yet it is the most neglected part of the human anatomy. A visit to various beaches during the bathing season will prove this to you. More than 75 percent of the people will probably have unsightly, weak, and flabby waistlines.

Proper development of the waist or abdominal muscles is of basic importance to everyone's health and strength, and has far-reaching beneficial effects upon the entire body. Proper development:

1. Prevents fat from accumulating about the middle; or reduces fat that has accumulated.
2. Is important in enabling the thin man to build up, because of its invigorating effect on the digestive organs.
3. Contributes markedly to the sculptural beauty of the body.
4. Prevents or overcomes constipation.
5. Protects against hernia (rupture) and visceral prolapse (sagging of the abdominal organs).
6. Assists in establishing and maintaining correct posture.
7. Is a great factor in developing bodily strength.

To understand how this affects the body, you must learn a little about the muscular formation of the abdomen, and its function.

From the base of the breastbone to the floor of the pelvis, the body is protected by a large membranous sheet of tissue in which four pairs of muscles are embedded—a perpendicular row of four on each side. The first three rows are somewhat square and of about equal size, and begin under the arch of the diaphragm, covering the stomach and the abdomen to about the line of the navel. The remaining two muscles are long, beginning at the navel and extending to the floor of the pubic bone. As they enter the groin they taper and lose considerable structure, and this makes them the weakest pair of muscles in the abdominal region. Their function is two-fold. Known as the *rectus abdominis,* they act in bending and straightening the body, and help to maintain an erect posture. Their secondary function is to promote health in the organs and stimulate the processes of the intestinal system. This is accomplished by the wavelike action of these muscles. With every bend, turn, and straightening of the body these muscles contract according to the extent of the movement. As they contract they corrugate in reeflike rows, which give them a washboard appearance. In the process of contraction they roll on the intestines with a pressure that creates a massaging effect and stimulates the process of evacuation. In this manner they coordinate with the muscular system that controls the channels of elimination. These are the *sphincter,* or circular compressor, muscles that surround the intestines for their entire length, providing the squeezing that moves the residue along the passages toward final evacuation.

Unfortunately, premature aging of the body becomes obvious with the first sign of increasing waist girth, which usually occurs in our early thirties and forties. Fat is our greatest enemy. Its corrosion destroys body tissue wherever it becomes deposited. Physical inactivity is the major cause of excess fat. Modern man sits in the streetcar, the subway, the auto, the office, and spends most of his spare time in the seated position. Before he knows it, his waist begins to deteriorate. This foreshortening of the body between the chest and the pelvis causes the waist muscles to lose their elasticity and contractile power, resulting in an outward bulge of the internal contents. The muscles, weakened by inactivity, yield to the pressure, allowing the unsightly bulge and unnatural sag, which ends in abdominal prolapse. He then becomes a candidate for many ailments that originate within the alimentary tract.

Finally, a fat-encumbered body is a hindrance to longevity. The statistics of life insurance companies show that the waistline is indeed the life line, and that every inch added to the abdomen after the age of forty takes off one year of life.

The importance of waistline development can never be overstated. Both fat men and thin men will benefit from it.

Surplus fat, especially abdominal fat, is almost always preventable or reducible; the means for accomplishing this need not be difficult or elaborate. A few minutes a day, given to exercises of the right kind, will soon transform a bulging waistline into a strong, firm, protective wall of muscle. An enormous improvement in health and all-around fitness is the result of this abdominal conditioning.

A strong, muscular waistline is equally desirable for a thin man. First, because of an increased breakdown of muscular tissue from exercise, the body needs more nourishment. Secondly, in response to that need, the vital organs work with increased power.

In promoting functional power in the digestive apparatus, too much attention can hardly be given to the muscles surrounding the trunk or body itself. Because of their proximity to the stomach, liver, and intestines, these muscles influence the organs in converting food into muscle and energy.

Above all, the obese should never practice the exercise generally advocated, where the subject touches his toes with his hands, bending over from an upright position with straight legs. It produces extreme body foreshortening, and is too severe on the back for those who have an inverted spine, which the obese usually do in various degrees whether they realize it or not.

Those with a distended or prolapsed stomach should also favor leg-raising exercises and the use of an inclined board. Those who are not afflicted with any of these conditions may perform the exercises in the regular manner, but when they come to the last exercise in this course they must follow the instructions implicitly to avoid bulking the abdominal contents against the muscle wall.

The young bodybuilder who exercises to obtain the fullest in abdominal development can follow this program exclusively. As he progresses in strength and development, he can use weights in the exercises that permit weights. In some exercises light dumbbells can be tied around the ankle or hitched onto the feet. Iron boots can be used, as they permit more weight, more exercises, and better control.

Muscular stimulation

The waistline must be muscularly stimulated in order to be properly conditioned and rebuilt. The right exercise is of paramount importance. When the outer or external muscles begin to contract and relax in exercising, the internal muscles perform the same work of contracting and relaxing. Some individuals turn to diet and massage in this rebuilding process, but although these measures are very helpful in eliminating fat and toxins and preventing further accumulation, they fall short of the objective.

Proper position for exercising

Corrective exercises are performed in the reverse position. That is, you should lie flat on your back or, better still, on an inclined board, with your feet slightly higher than your head. This allows your stomach and abdomen to spread out naturally. When you lift your legs toward your body, the abdominal contents fall inward and away from the muscular wall, thereby allowing full and unrestricted functioning of the muscles from the groin to the chest. More varied and advanced exercises can be practiced once this objective is achieved. Women who, following childbirth, neglect their waist region also fall in the category of having a distended waistline.

When you practice the exercises in this course your abdominal muscles will become completely developed, as will the muscles of your sides, the small of your back, and your hips. This does *not* mean that your hips will become larger. The buttock muscles are heavily supplied with fatty tissue in men as well as women. Exercise will reduce the excess fatty content of the hips just as it will reduce the abdomen or any other part of the body. Your hips will become more compact and shapely. Your vigor will be improved, and organic functions will acquire new energy as they are freed from the clogging of excess fat. New vitality will impregnate all the tissues of the body, and life again will be worth living. You will take pride in your improved shapeliness, and youth will return to you.

Training, not straining

The following exercises must be performed regularly and in graduated amounts. The object is to *train* and not to *strain*. Allow at least two hours to elapse after eating before exercising, to allow your body time for digestion. Breathe deeply and naturally at all times. It is best to exhale with the effort and inhale as you return to the starting position. Wear as little clothing as possible to allow for freedom of motion. Watch your posture: sit straight, walk erect, and do not slouch over. Your faithful performance of the exercises will be rewarding—you will feel and look years younger.

Abdominal Exercises

Group A

Exercise 1. Lie flat on your back with your hands under your hips and your legs stretched out straight. Slowly draw up the knee of one leg as close to your body as possible. Thrust your leg straight out from this position, without allowing the heel to touch the floor. Repeat the exercise with your other leg; alternate legs. Keep your toes pointed and force your knees well back, keeping your legs in as straight a line as possible. Exhale while drawing your knee up and inhale while extending your leg.

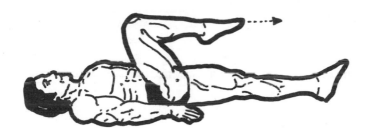

Abdomen Exercise A1

Repeat 12 times with each leg and gradually work up to 24 repetitions.

Exercise 2. Assume the same position as for exercise 1. Slowly raise one leg toward your head, while breathing out and drawing in your abdomen. Breathe in as you lower your leg to the floor, then repeat with your other leg. Keep your legs rigid and your toes pointed throughout the exercise, and raise your leg as far toward your head as you can.

Repeat eight times with each leg and gradually work up to 24 repetitions. Excellent for lower abdomen and pelvis muscles.

Exercise 3. Assume the same position as for exercise 1. Without bending your knees, raise both legs toward your head as far as possible, breathing out and drawing in your abdomen as you do so. Return to starting position inhaling. Keep your legs straight and your toes pointed throughout the exercise. Gradually learn not to allow your heels to touch the floor between leg raises.

Repeat 12 times and gradually work up to 24 repetitions. Splendid for your lower abdominal muscles.

Exercise 4. Assume the same position as for exercise 1. Make sure to keep your hands under your hips to prevent your body from rolling. Raise both feet about a foot off the floor. Kick your feet up and down past each other in alternate fashion. Keep your legs straight and do not allow your heels to touch the floor. Breathe in and out evenly, and use short kicks as your feet pass one another.

Practice this exercise 12 times with each leg. Add two repetitions at every third practice session until you are making 36 kicks with each leg. (Thirty-six is the limit of repetitions for this exercise.)

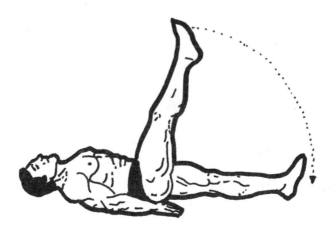

Abdomen Exercise A2

Exercise 5. Sit on the floor with your hands clasped behind your neck as shown in the drawing. Twist or rotate at the waist as far to the right as possible, bending forward as you do so, then twist to the left in the same manner. Breathe in and out naturally. Carry the twist to each side slowly and completely, almost touching your opposite knee with your elbow.

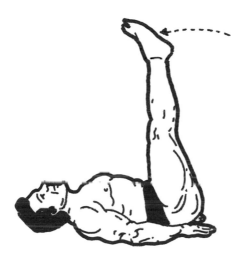

Abdomen Exercise A3

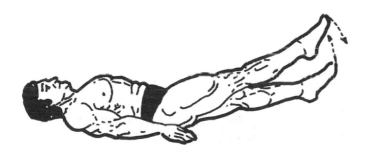

Abdomen Exercise A4

Repeat 12 twists to each side and gradually work up to 36 twists to each side. Excellent for the abdominals and side waist muscles.

Exercise 6. Assume the same position as for exercise 1. Draw both knees back over your abdomen as shown in the drawing, keeping your knees together and toes pointed. Extend both legs fully forward without letting your feet touch the floor. Exhale while flexing your legs, and inhale while extending them. Keep your hands under your buttocks to keep your body from rolling.

Repeat nine times and gradually work up to 36 repetitions.

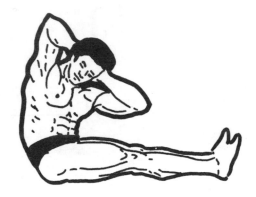

Abdomen Exercise A5

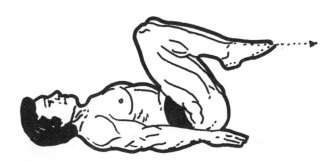

Exercise 7. Assume the same position as for exercise 1. Raise your legs to a right angle with your body, and describe a circle with each leg. Breathe in and out naturally.

Make eight circles with each leg, gradually working up to 24 circles; maintain this count.

Exercise 8. Lie prone, with your arms and legs fully extended. Exhaling, throw both arms forward and rise to a

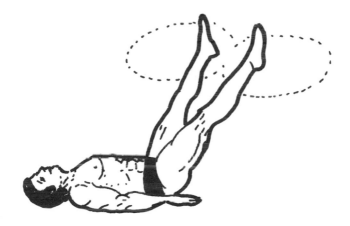

Abdomen Exercise A7

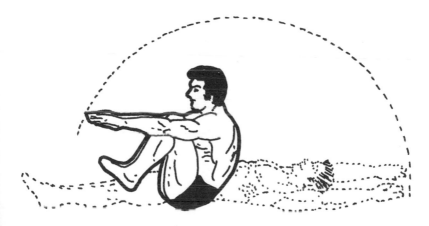

Abdomen Exercise A8

sitting position, bringing both knees to your chest at the same time, as illustrated. Hold this position, and push both legs out at full length without touching the floor, then bring them back to your chest. Exhale while returning to the starting position.

Learn to coordinate your movements, bringing your upper body forward and flexing your legs towards your chest simultaneously. Exhale both while sitting up and while returning to the starting position.

Repeat nine times and gradually work up to 24. This is an excellent exercise for developing all of the abdominal and groin muscles.

Exercise 9. Lie flat on the floor with your feet under a heavy object (such as the edge of a dresser), with your hands clasped behind your head. Sit up, pulling your head forward with your arms as you do so, and try to touch your knees with your elbows. Breathe out completely as you sit up and bend forward. Inhale slowly and deeply as you return to the starting position. Do not strain, but bring your head and elbows as close to your knees as possible. Pull your waist in as you exhale.

Repeat 12 times and slowly work up to 24 repetitions;

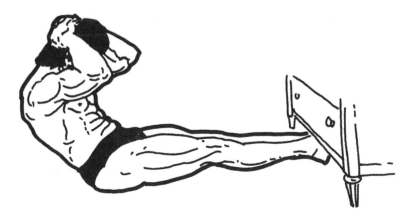

Abdomen Exercise A9

maintain this limit. After many months of training, a light weight can be held against the back of your neck to increase the effort for further strength and development.

Exercise 10. Lie on your back with your arms fully extended. Breathe out and quickly raise your hands over your head, and at the same time kick up with your legs held straight in an effort to touch your fingers and toes as shown. Hold this position for a second, if possible. Breathe in as you return to the starting position. Learn to coordinate this movement, kicking your legs and raising your upper body at the same time.

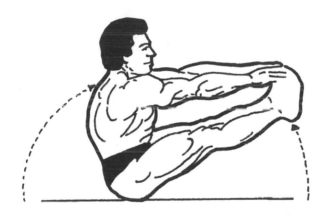

Abdomen Exercise A10

Repeat 12 times and slowly work up to 24 repetitions; maintain this limit. This exercise is excellent for the abdominal, hip, and buttock muscles. The speed involved in this movement will help keep the waist muscles supple.

Exercise 11. Stand upright with your feet spaced comfortably apart. With your right hand, hold a dumbbell at arm's length overhead. Bend over to the left, bending your left knee and touching your left foot with your left hand. Return to the erect position and repeat six times. Change the dumbbell over to your left hand and repeat the exercise on the right. Be sure to keep the dumbbell at arm's length throughout the exercise.

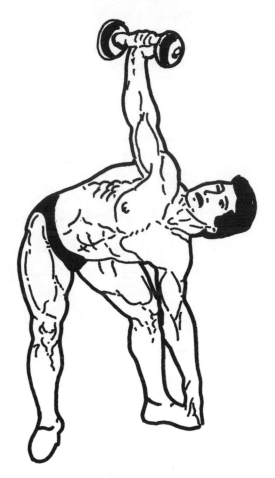

Abdomen Exercise A11

Repeat six times and gradually work up to 18 repetitions, then add five pounds to the dumbbell and start over with six repetitions.

Exercise 12. Stand erect with the dumbbells held on your shoulders. The whole idea of this exercise is to press a dumbbell overhead alternately with each arm as illustrated, while bending your trunk straight from side to side. Breathe naturally and always bend directly to the side. Keep an erect posture and do not slump at any time.

Repeat 12 times with each arm, gradually working up to 24 repetitions with each arm. Then add five pounds to each bell and begin again with the original count of 12. This overhead pressing and side bending exercise is one of the best movements for the side waist muscles, and also influences back, shoulder, and arm development.

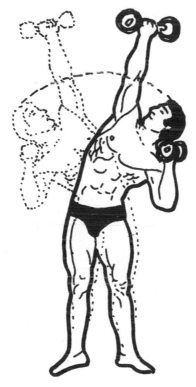

Abdomen Exercise A12

Advanced Abdominal Exercises

Group B

Exercise 1. Sit erect with your elbows clasped behind your head, and then bend backward as shown in the illustration. Inhale on the backward movement and exhale while returning to your starting position. Start with nine repetitions and gradually work up to 18 counts. This exercise is excellent for the complete abdominal structure, groin, and lower back.

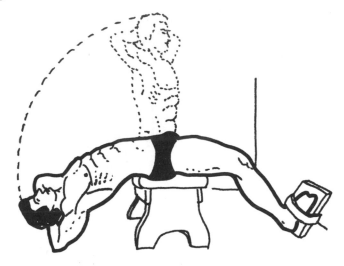

Abdomen Exercise B1

Exercise 2. The reverse sit-up. Study the illustration carefully. With your hips extending over the stool in the position shown and your legs straight, raise and lower your trunk until your back muscles are tired. Exhale and relax your muscles when lowering your body. Inhale on coming back to the starting position and at the same time arch your back, lifting your head as high as possible, keeping your elbows firmly backward, and tensing all the muscles of your back from head to toes.

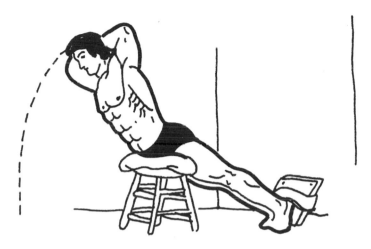

Abdomen Exercise B2

Repeat nine times (or until you are tired) and gradually work up to 18 counts. This exercise is excellent for all the back muscles, the loins, and for coordinating the waist musculature.

Exercise 3. The side sit-up. Study the illustration carefully and note how the body is set directly sideways and the crossed position of the feet. Alternately raise and lower your body in exactly the same manner shown in the illustration. Exhale on lowering your body as far as possible and inhale on returning to the starting position, raising your body as high as possible. Change to the opposite side of your body and repeat. Repeat nine times and gradually work up to 18 counts. This exercise is excellent for developing the external and internal oblique muscles at the sides of the waist, the erector spine muscles of the back, and the latissimus dorsi muscles which are the broadest muscles of the back.

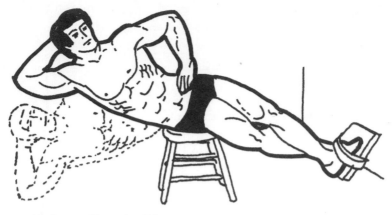

Abdomen Exercise B3

Note: It would be best to use a stool with a cushion as shown in the illustrations, with your feet secured under a bureau, couch, or other heavy piece of furniture. A board attached securely to the wall and the floor at an angle of about 45 degrees, with a leather belting running around it is even better.

These exercises can be made more advanced by holding your arms overhead and going through the movements as described, or holding a weight to your head while going through the movements.

Advanced Abdominal Exercises

Group C

Exercises 1, 2, 3, 4, 6, and 7 of Group A can be performed with iron health boots. Turn to page 103 and check the instructions given for iron or aluminum health boots. The movements of the exercises are exactly the same, but the boots allow greater stress to be put on the abdominal muscles, and thus enhance their development.

The inclined or slant board, which can be purchased at

any sport or health-fitness shop, is an excellent piece of equipment for abdominal exercises. Movements from the simplest to the most advanced exercises can be performed on the slant board.

In the sit-up or upper body movements, a weight or dumbbell can be held at chest level. For greater stress, the same weight can be held behind the neck.

It is most important that you perform the exercises perfectly as outlined in the instructions. Always exhale on raising your upper body or legs toward the center of your body. Inhale on relaxing and returning to the starting position. Above all, never strain.

Put Power into Your Legs

Our health and general physical efficiency depends on our legs to an appreciable extent. This does not mean that disproportionate legs always typify an unhealthy body, but it does mean that better legs contribute greatly to better health. Physical endurance, the vital factor in body efficiency, is related to the amount of power possessed in the legs. The heart, lungs, and blood stream receive their greatest stimulation from the action of the legs. If the legs are healthily and strongly constructed, the stimulation given to the body is vitally healthful.

The legs make a very interesting study. They are full of mechanical links and levers and have a great deal to do with bodily health.

How many people know that they are sick when they are constantly complaining about cold legs or cold feet, when their skin is crinkled up like goose flesh, or when their legs are swollen and flabby? Not many, but they are, and the main causes for this are poor muscular structure, stagnant circulation, and impoverished blood.

The two important points to be explained concerning these danger signals are that the legs contain some of the largest muscles in the body, and being far removed from the heart, they require more action to stir up their circulation. The legs are also part of the body where the blood flows contrary to gravity.

Good legs are as essential to a person as steel pillars are to a building. A good pair of underpinnings usually indicates a powerful hip formation, and enhances vitality.

86

In order to walk upright, carry, or lift, we must resist the gravity. Therefore it is only natural that the legs, like any other material foundation, should be the strongest part of our physical architecture.

Knees give way under the pressure of a back load too often, and this is more likely when a strong back is paired with weak legs. I have seen some men, powerful looking above the waist, fold up under a shoulder load.

The legs, coupled with the hips and buttocks (which cooperate in almost every leg exercise) make up nearly half the muscular bulk of the body. The actions of these muscles are diversified, and it follows that the movements used to develop them fully must also be widely varied.

The important muscles of your legs

It may surprise you to learn that one lower leg has thirty bones, not including those of the pelvis. Naturally, these bones are all subject to movement, and this can only be accomplished by muscles.

It is amazing to find, as you go from the hip to the sole of the foot, how numerous the muscles are and what an influence better leg construction has on your upper body, particularly your organs.

Something else that is important to your health takes place in the great bones of your legs. The red corpuscles of your body are manufactured in the marrow of your bones. These corpuscles are the nucleus of your blood stream. And more red corpuscles means a richer blood stream.

No matter how strong your upper body is, your legs will not be able to back up your bodily effort unless they are also strong.

The most important muscle in the thigh is the *vastus internus*—the inside thigh member of the *quadriceps femoris,* directly above the inside of your knee. The great importance of this muscle lies in its rocklike power in locking your knee.

High up in the pelvis, a muscle, the *tensor fascia lata,* helps to complete that beautiful sweeping outside curve seen on the well-developed thigh.

The other important muscle that originates in the pelvis and fastens below the knee is the *sartorius.* This is the longest muscle in the body and is a very interesting and unusual part of your thigh construction.

The muscles that draw your legs together from the knees-spread-apart position are the *gracilis.* Hollowed-out inner thighs are the result of poor gracilis development.

The largest muscle is the one that bulks on the front of the thigh; it is known as the *quadriceps femoris,* meaning "four-headed thigh muscle." The *rectus femoris* is the largest of these, and lies directly on the front of the thigh. The action of this muscle straightens your leg.

The other important thigh muscles are located at the back of your thigh: the *biceps,* or "twin-headed muscles." Actually, there are three muscles in this group and they are referred to for study as the hamstring muscles. Their action is to flex the knee (that is, to bend it), and also to raise the leg backward.

The *soleus* muscle is connected to the *gastrocnemius* muscle. It begins where the gastrocnemius leaves off and joins the *Achilles tendon.* Right under the gastrocnemius (as you look at a well-shaped calf from the back) you will notice a body of tissue which tapers in a broad triangle toward the ankle; this is mainly the *soleus.* Toward the ankle, the Achilles tendon is more evident.

Leg Exercises

Group A

Exercise 1. Stand perfectly erect with your hands cupped on your hips. Slowly rise as high as possible on your toes, maintaining an erect posture and balance, then return to the starting position. Keep your knees locked throughout the movement. If you find it difficult to balance properly, rest the fingertips of one hand lightly on a chair back. Remember to maintain an erect posture at all times. If you get a cramp in your foot or calf, relieve it with massage.

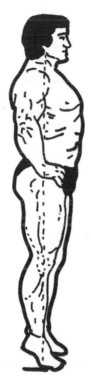

Leg Exercise A1—Body-Weight Lift on the Toes

Repeat 16 times and gradually work up to 32 counts in perfect form. Once you have perfected your performance in this exercise, you can vary it by using one leg. Rise on one foot, bending the other leg at the knee. Alternate legs and perform exactly as above, maintaining your balance. Excellent for the entire leg, from buttocks to toes.

Exercise 2. Stand erect with your feet about six inches apart, and your hands on your hips. Raise your right leg to the right angle position shown (position 1), pointing your toes directly forward. Next bend your foot backward on the ankle (position 2). Slowly bend your knee backward and upward as far as possible, pointing your toes toward the floor, keeping the heel of your foot close to your buttocks (position 3). Return to starting position.

Repeat until tired. Alternate with left leg, and practice slowly and exactly. Splendid for the development of the thigh biceps muscle. When the toes are forcibly pointed as shown, the gastrocnemius muscles of the calf are brought into play.

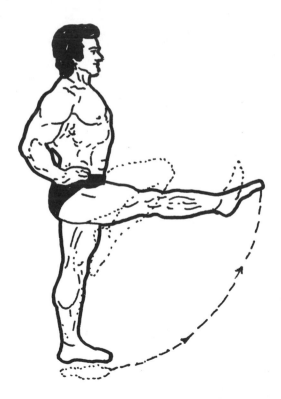

Leg Exercise A2

Exercise 3. Stand erect, placing your hand on a table in order to control balance. Raise your outside leg directly sideways as far as possible without bending your body in any direction. From this position, turn your foot in all directions—up, down, and around. Return to starting position.

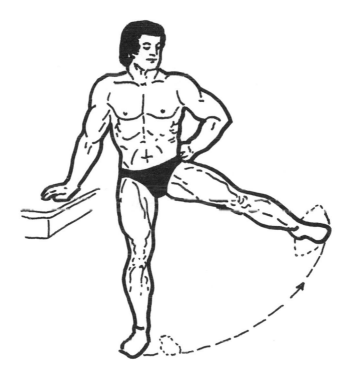

Leg Exercise A3

Repeat six times, then repeat with other leg. Gradually work up to 18 repetitions with each leg. Splendid for the outside muscles of the thighs, known as the tensor fascia lata, which fill out the thighs with fullness and contour when fully developed.

Exercise 4. Stand perfectly erect and bend your knee as illustrated. Place a towel or cord around the top of your foot. Slowly pull upward with both hands, resisting with your lower leg or calf, until the heel is brought close to your buttocks, as illustrated in Fig. 2. Do not strain. Alternate legs.

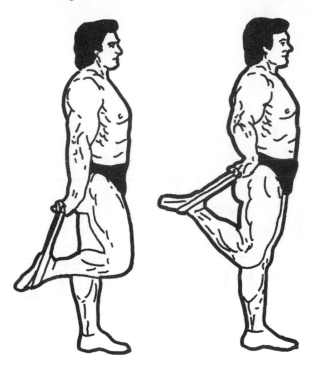

Leg Exercise A4

Start with six repetitions and gradually work up to 12 counts with each leg. This exercise is excellent for the ankle, calf, knee, back of thigh, and buttock muscles.

Exercise 5. Stand perfectly erect with your feet about ten inches apart. Lower your body into the knee bend position, and at the same time bring your arms directly forward, without raising your heels from the floor. Exhale going down, and inhale completely while returning to the starting position.

Practice this movement 12 times and gradually work up to 24 counts. The squat not only develops the thigh muscles and the muscles of the shins, but also has a beneficial effect on the abdominal organs. The good effect on the lungs and chest muscles is induced by deep breathing.

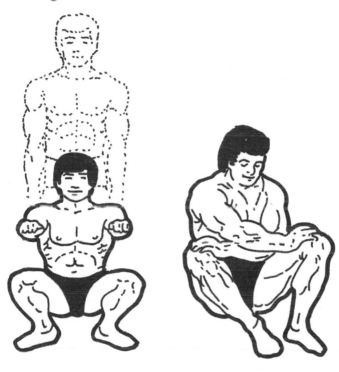

Leg Exercise A5—The Squat   Leg Exercise A6

Note: In this exercise it will be necessary to incline your body slightly forward from the hips in order to maintain good balance. Otherwise observe all directions given for performing the knee bend (exercise 8 of this group).

Exercise 6. Assume a sitting position on the floor. Cross your arms, placing your right hand against the inside of your left knee. Hold your knees fairly close together, and draw your heels up towards your buttocks. With all your power, push each hand against the inside of your thigh, and as you do so, resist the pressure of your hands by squeezing in with your knees. The object of this exercise is to spread your knees apart as much as you can with hand pressure while resisting with your thigh muscles. When your knees have been spread apart as far as they will go, slip your hands across your knees so that your hands are now pulling your knees inward. Forcibly try to pull your knees together with your hands and resist the effort with your thighs.

Repeat nine times in each direction, and gradually work up to 18 counts in each direction.

Note: In the first part of this exercise you push your knees apart and in the second stage you pull them together, but in each movement you resist with your legs. Excellent for the muscles along the inside and outside of the thigh.

Exercise 7. Stand erect with your hands on your hips. Stand with your feet well apart and your toes turned in as far as possible. From this awkward position, begin to bend at the knees and descend into a semi-sitting position, bringing your knees slowly and forcibly together. Return to the starting position.

Repeat nine times; gradually work up to 24 repetitions. Excellent for bringing the muscles not employed in the knee bend or the full squat into play. The thigh and calf muscles, as well as the knees and ankles, are involved in a different action.

Note: It is not necessary to make a complete squat. The movement as illustrated is all that is necessary—the knee action at the conclusion of the exercise does the trick.

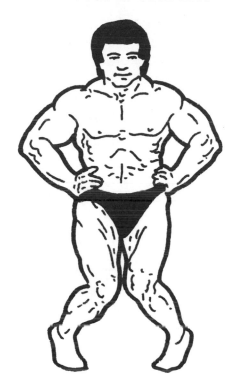

Leg Exercise A7—The Semi-Squat

Exercise 8. Stand perfectly erect, heels together, toes pointed outward, and arms at sides as shown in the illustration. Lower your body by bending at the knees, bringing your arms forward to shoulder level and raising your heels off the floor at the same time. Return to the upright position, bringing your arms back to your sides. Maintain good posture and balance throughout the movement.

Practice this exercise 12 times and gradually work up to 24 repetitions. The movement can be varied by keeping the heels close together or wide apart. Excellent for the front, inside, and part of the outside of the thighs and the groin muscles.

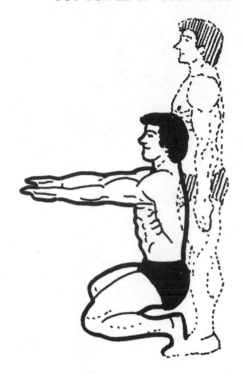

Leg Exercise A8—The Knee Bend

Leg Exercises

Group B

Exercise 1. Stand erect, holding a dumbbell in each hand. Place your toes and the balls of your feet on a block of wood about two inches high, resting your heels on the floor. Slowly raise your body, without bending your knees, until you are standing entirely on your toes and the balls of your feet. Breathe in as you raise your body and out as you lower your heels to the floor. Keep your body perfectly erect throughout the movement. Note the dotted line in the illustration which projects the body balance, and let your calf muscles perform the exercise.

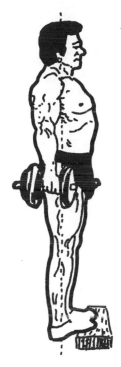

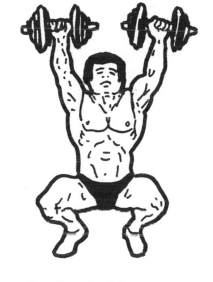

Leg Exercise B1   Leg Exercise B2

Repeat 12 times. Add one repetition at every third practice session until 24 counts are made, then add five pounds to each bell and start over with the original count.

Exercise 2. Stand erect with your feet well apart, and the dumbbells held overhead. Keeping an erect posture, squat down, raising your body on your toes as shown. Then slowly rise on your toes back to the starting position, maintaining the dumbbells at arm's length overhead. Breathe out while squatting and inhale while returning to the starting position. Keep an erect posture and balance throughout. Do not hold your breath and do not strain.

Practice six times. Gradually work up to 12 repetitions, then add 2½ pounds to each bell and start over with six repetitions. This exercise is excellent for the entire leg structure, including the hips and the lower back musculature.

Exercise 3. Stand erect with your feet spread well apart. Place the barbell behind your neck and across your shoulders as shown in the illustration. From this position, rise up on your toes, breathe in, and lower your body to the position shown by bending your knees. Breathe out as you return to the starting position, using the power of your legs to raise your body. Keep your back straight throughout the movement.

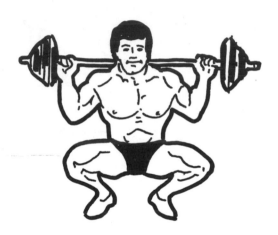

Leg Exercise B3

Repeat nine times. Add one repetition at every third practice session until 18 counts are reached, then add ten pounds to the barbell and start over with nine repetitions. This exercise is excellent for all of the leg muscles.

Exercise 4. Stand erect and place a barbell across the back of your neck. Place a stool, chair, or small bench directly in front of you as shown. Place one foot on the bench, and using only your leg strength, step up on the stool with your other leg. Do not strain. Now step down and repeat in exactly the same manner using your other leg. Keep erect at all times. Breathe in and out naturally, and use only your leg strength.

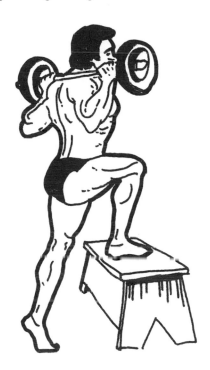

Leg Exercise B4

Repeat nine times with each leg. Add one repetition at every third practice session until you can perform 18 counts. Then add 10 pounds to the barbell and start over with nine repetitions. This exercise is excellent for the hips and thighs.

Exercise 5. Stand perfectly erect with the barbell across your shoulders. Now place your left leg about 12 inches forward, as shown in Fig. 1. From this position, begin to bend your knees, pushing your left knee as far forward as possible until you are balanced on your toes in the position shown in Fig. 2. Without moving the position of your feet, return to the erect starting position. Your feet *must* remain in the same position throughout the movement. Breathe in as you squat and out as you return to the starting position. Use a weight within your control in order to secure balance and proper movement.

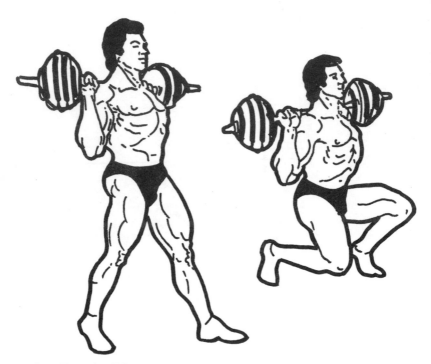

Leg Exercise B5

Repeat eight times with each leg. Gradually increase the repetitions until you can perform 16 movements perfectly with each leg, then add ten pounds to the bar and start over with eight repetitions. Splendid for the hips, thighs, and calves.

Exercise 6. With a barbell resting on your shoulders, stand erect, take a deep breath, and slowly bend your knees and squat down to the position shown, breathing out on your way down. Take another deep breath and rise to an erect position, keeping your back as flat as possible throughout the exercise. Many bodybuilders handle too heavy a weight and perform the exercise incorrectly—therefore most of the benefit is lost. They usually handle a very heavy weight, drop into the squat position, and rise on the rebound. This should never be done if you want to develop your leg muscles. It is better to handle a lighter weight and perform the movement correctly, concentrating on your legs.

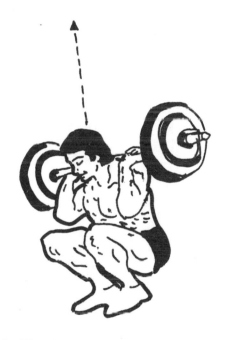

Leg Exercise B6—The Full Squat

Repeat this exercise nine times. Add one count at every third practice session until 18 counts are made, then add ten pounds to the barbell and start over from the count of nine.

Exercise 7. Skipping is a great leg developer, but more important, skipping promotes endurance and energy in the leg muscles. Muscles must have endurance in order to be strong.

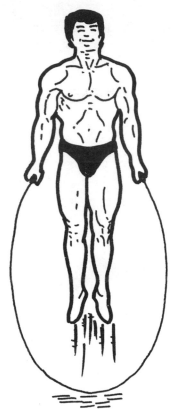

Leg Exercise B7

Exercise 8. The number circle will test your leg strength, energy, and endurance. Start in a semi-squat position in the center of the ring, and then bound forward, backward, and sideways in all directions without stopping. This promotes a better control of balance, a quick eye, and quick-acting muscles.

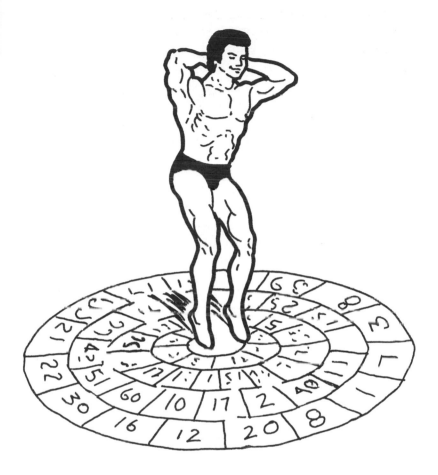

Leg Exercise B8—The Number Circle

Special Advanced Leg Exercises

Group C

Iron or aluminum boots can be used for all advanced leg exercises. This equipment can be strapped to your feet as roller skates are. The exercises can be progressively graduated by adding weight plates to the existing weight attachments.

Most of the exercises listed in "Trim Your Waistline" can be performed with the iron boots, namely exercises 1, 2, 3, 4, 6, and 7. The hips and buttocks are also greatly aided in the development by these special advanced leg movements. These exercises must be performed perfectly. This means "no cheating" if the exercises are to be done correctly. If you cannot perform the exercises with perfect balance, you are not prepared for the advanced leg movements.

At first, use your boots alone, or use only that weight which will enable you to perform 12 correct movements and follow out the instructions accordingly. Add one repetition on every third practice night until 18 counts are reached; then add two or three pounds to the boots and start over from the original count of 12.

Advancement would consist of adding weight to the boots and duplicating the routine. This is termed another "set."

Maintain good posture and balance at all times, never hold your breath, and breathe naturally.

Iron boot exercises

Study the illustrations carefully. If you cannot perform 12 counts correctly, then practice until you are tired, and gradually work up to 12 counts. Thereafter, follow the instructions as previously stated.

Exercise 1. Stand erect. Raise your right knee as high as possible toward your chest, then lower slowly to starting position and repeat. At the conclusion of 12 counts, repeat with your left leg in exactly the same manner.

Exercise 2. Stand erect. Raise your right knee to a right angle position. Pause, then extend your leg directly forward. Bring your leg back to the right-angle position, lower slowly to starting position and repeat. Repeat with your left leg in exactly the same manner.

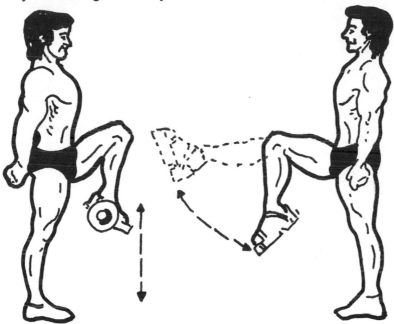

Leg Exercise C1   Leg Exercise C2

Exercise 3. Stand erect. Bend your right leg at the knee, lifting your lower leg backward as high as possible, pointing your knee toward the floor as illustrated. Return slowly to starting position. Repeat with your left leg in exactly the same manner.

Exercise 4. Stand erect. Raise your right leg forward as high as possible. Lower slowly and repeat. Keep your leg as straight as possible throughout the movement. Perform in exactly the same manner with your left leg.

Exercise 5. Stand erect. Raise your right leg directly sideways as high as possible, keeping your leg straight. Return slowly to starting position and repeat. Repeat with your left leg in exactly the same manner. It is important

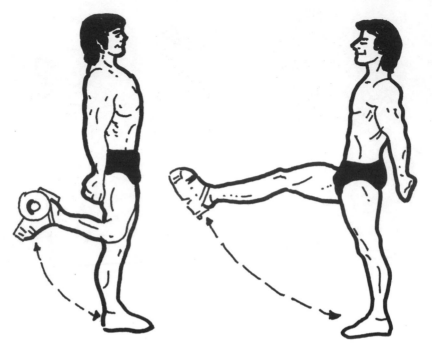

Leg Exercise C3   Leg Exercise C4

that you move only your leg, without using or twisting your upper body; this goes for all leg movements.

Exercise 6. Sit erect on a bench or the edge of a table. Raise the lower part of your right leg directly forward until the leg is perfectly straight. Lower slowly to starting position and repeat the desired number of counts. Follow through with your left leg in exactly the same manner. For variation, you can exercise both legs at the same time in this position.

Exercise 7. Lying flat on your back, raise both legs to a right angle with your body. Keeping your legs perfectly straight, slowly part them as far as possible sideways. Pause, and then bring them back together at the starting position and repeat. This is an excellent movement for the muscles along the inside of your thighs.

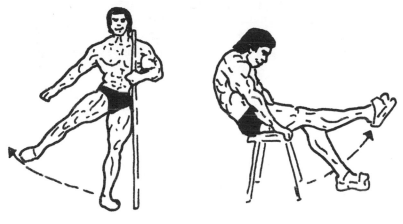

Leg Exercise C5   Leg Exercise C6

Exercise 8. This is known as the "bicycle" exercise. Lie flat on your back, and pull your feet up overhead so that your body rests on your shoulders and upper back. Support your body by gripping your hips with your hands

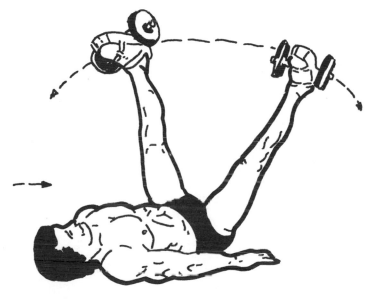

Leg Exercise C7

and putting your weight on your elbows, as shown. Lower one leg and as you begin to lower your second leg push the first one upward and overhead. Continue revolving your legs in this manner, similar to riding a bicycle.

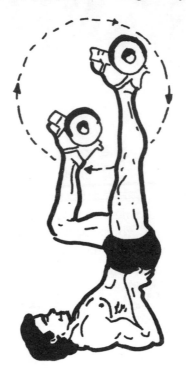

Leg Exercise C8

Exercise 9. Lie face down with your legs stretched out in a straight line with your body. From this position, bend your lower legs back to a right-angle position and as far as possible toward your hips without straining. Lower and repeat.

Iron boot exercises 10, 11, 12, 13, 14, and 15 are exactly the same as exercises 1, 2, 3, 4, 6, and 7 in "Trim Your Waistline."

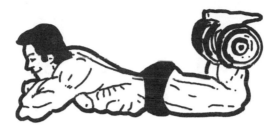

Leg Exercise C9

Important points to observe

Make sure that your boots are securely attached to your feet when exercising. Strong, well-formed legs will only come about with faithful and consistent practice. All of the exercises given should not be done in a single workout, but you should practice three or four of them in one excrcise session. In the following session you can choose three or four more, and so forth, until you have practiced all of the exercises. Carefully read every word of the exercise descriptions and study the illustrations closely before attempting them, as your success depends on the proper application and execution of the exercises. Remember at all times that your objective is to train, not to strain.

Strong Bodies
Need Strong Spines

A strong spine makes for good health and a strong body. A weak spine causes sacroiliac trouble, spinal curvatures, misplaced vertebrae, and many other painful troubles. Every bodybuilder and athlete needs a powerful spine.

Building a strong spine is the key to building a strong body. The spinal column, with its associated muscles and ligaments, and the 26 bones attached to it directly and indirectly, gives support, strength, and flexibility to the rest of the body.

Spinal strength is necessary to allow your body to function vigorously. Proper alignment of the spine allows the vital organs to maintain their normal position for efficient functioning. If your spine has trouble maintaining a proper position, these vital organs begin to sag and become cramped. The spinal nerves, which emanate to every organ and part of the body and distribute impulses are interfered with if pressure is exerted on them. This interference can disturb the body; a weak spine carries a multitude of ills. Disturbances of the vital organs and various types of nervous disorders have their origin in weakness of the spine.

At the close of a working day you have often said to yourself that you felt as though your back were broken. It ached with a dull throb that took all the pep out of you, and when you bent over, you were forced to struggle back to an erect position by pushing on your knees with your hands. Your hips felt as stiff as a board. Walking was wearying. When you got home you "flopped into a chair" or onto the couch like a broken hinge, and, worst of all, this gave you little relief. You said you were getting old and that you felt "rotten." You felt rotten all right, but this is not exactly a sign that you are becoming prematurely old. Fatigue had really caused what you were feeling but you did not understand this.

Your spine is composed of a series of bony segments, named *vertebrae*. They pyramid on top of each other from the floor of the *pelvis,* which is the space between your hip bones. The vertebrae in your pelvic region are the most heavily constructed, and they gradually taper in size as they ascend your spinal shaft. These bony segments graduate from rigidity to a certain flexibility, and the apex of pliability is reached in what you know best as the "small of the back." This is where physical strain is imposed in movements of bending or twisting from the normal erect posture. It is also here that your spine is least protected. This section is called the "fulcrum" of your body because the major physical strain is registered here. All other muscular parts of your body are supported by fixed, unbendable bones which move only in joints. No matter how tired the muscles surrounding the fixed bones become, the bones are never affected. Not so with the spine in the small of your back, properly termed the *lumbar region*—a name you will recognize because of its similarity to *lumbago,* a form of back strain invariably caused by fatigue. The lumbar region is the "hinge of the body," and unless the muscles composing the small of your back are well conditioned, abnormal strain is imposed on your spine, causing a weariness which makes the effort of carrying your body erect a little more strenuous toward the end of the day.

How your spine is thrown out of alignment

If you could register the thousands of bends, turns, and twists that you perform daily at the apex of your trunk, you would realize what a punishment these muscles take. It is not hard to understand how the spine is thrown out of alignment when the muscles become too tired to support the vertebrae in the lumbar region. However, this is not as common, nor as dangerous, as a subtle condition which constantly occurs in this area. To help you understand this better, let me explain that the backbone is built to meet the pressure of body weight forced down on each of the vertebrae, particularly in the lumbar region. To offset the pressure, nature provided gristly pads between your spinal vertebrae and these act like shock absorbers. These pads are thickest in the lumbar region because they receive the greatest pressure. The pads become flattened out from constant pressure by the end of the day, and when you are engaged in manual work, lifting objects of any sort, the pads are compressed even more.

When your back muscles tire, the vertebrae lack complete natural support and are in danger of being tipped more than normal. Worse still, your vertebrae can be deprived of part of their natural seating in the cups of their mates, which makes displacement of a vertebra a simple matter. When this happens, either the nerve branching from the side of the vertebra, or its feeder, can become pinched. The muscles in that particular spot are then deprived of their dynamic nerve energy.

Rejuvenating your vitality depends on how you cooperate with nature

In the evening, and during sleep, the pads between your vertebrae adjust themselves to normal if they can—but that again is up to you. Recuperation manifests itself during your sleep, to your best advantage, consequently rejuvenating yourself depends upon how you cooperate with nature, in keeping your body tuned to build that abundant measure of energy necessary to meet the mental and physical emergencies of the next day, and every other day during your life.

A strong erect spine is the foundation of the entire physical structure. The person with this type of spine manifests health and strength. He carries an air of confidence—not the defeatist attitude of those individuals who are bent over and doubled up. Proper internal functioning allows the strong-spined individual to have that amount of organic vigor which is a part of abounding health.

The strength and flexibility of the spine depend on the working efficiency of the spinal muscles. All the muscles of the back and spine are interrelated and correlated and work for the good of the entire spinal structure by giving it the necessary support, strength, and motion.

Proper attention to the development of all these muscles is one of the most important factors in molding a strong back and a healthy spine. The only way it can be made strong is to use it. Proper exercise will do a great deal toward building a strong, erect spine and improving the health and vitality of the body.

When you exercise the spine, you are not only promoting greater flexibility and strength, but you are stimulating the delicate spinal cord and nerves. Constant movement of the muscles and ligaments produces a massagelike effect on the nerve structures, and this increases their activity. Circulation of the blood is improved and toxins are removed. In short, we must work through the muscles to stimulate the health and strength of the spine.

Practically speaking, there are only three groups of muscles on the back that need be considered. These groups govern the lesser groups, so whatever exercise is done to improve the three groups will improve the lesser muscles as well.

The first group are the *trapezius* muscles. Together, the pair of the trapezius muscles is shaped like a trapezium. They aid in all of the functions of the back, such as shrugging the shoulders, bracing back the shoulders, and maintaining the erect position of the head. Their major bulk is in the caplike formation across the shoulders at the base of the neck. If you clasp your hands tightly together behind your back and bring your shoulder blades together you will see these muscles bunching up.

They run down from the base of the head toward the points of the shoulders, and gradually taper off down the spine like spears. They have a triple insertion and are very capable muscles. Although they do not have a great deal to do with widening the back, they thicken it and promote great nerve vitality.

The second group are the *latissimus dorsi* muscles, which are the broad back muscles. They cover the majority of the back, and run from the lower back to the shoulder blades where they taper off into a powerful tendon fastened onto the *humerus* bone (the bone of the upper arm). These muscles have the most to do with increasing the width of the back. They are very powerful muscles and due to their scapular insertion (attachment to the shoulder blades) are capable of spreading their range.

The third group are the *spinae erector* muscles, the muscles that erect the spine, sometimes known as the spinal column or the "column of Hercules." The many names illustrate the importance of these muscles. They are probably the most important in back muscular formation. If they are weak, then your spine is exposed to all the troubles that can affect it, from spinal displacement to lumbago. These muscles control the turning, bending, and erection of the body. The important thing to learn is always to keep your back as straight as humanly possible. When the back is rounded at the waistline—the lumbar region—the spinae erector muscles flatten and do not give the necessary support to the spine. Since the lumbar area is the weakest section of the spinal chain, every effort should be made to secure the best possible muscular protection.

Special attention to the third group will give an ample coating of muscular armor for this purpose, and will also broaden the small of the back, giving the spine a firmer foundation on the lower back.

These muscles appear as a column of thick rope on each side of the spine, and form a channel or groove in which the spine is engulfed. They appear bulkiest in the small of the back, but they continue all the way up the spine to final insertion in the base of the head. They submerge under all the other muscles at about the line of the floating ribs.

These things properly noted and indexed in the mind, let us consider how best to develop these muscles.

Exercise Program

Basic freehand program

The average person can practice the following exercises to advantage. They can be performed at any time. As always, it's best to wait at least one or two hours after eating before exercising. Wear as little clothing as possible to allow for freedom of motion. See that you are breathing fresh air at all times—in other words, there should be proper ventilation.

Group A

Exercise 1. Lie face downward on a flat table or on the floor, and clasp your hands behind your back. Now raise your head and shoulders. Return to starting position. Vary and twist the shoulders from right to left.

Exercise 2. Same as exercise 1, only this time you raise your legs, first the left and then the right. Then raise both at the same time as far upward as you can.

Exercise 3. Lie on your back with your head on a pillow, and your fingers interlaced over your abdomen. Raise up to form a "bridge" with your head and heels. Then twist your shoulders—left down and left up. Do not strain. If this is too difficult at first, just bridge up and down without twisting until your neck becomes stronger.

Exercise 4. Sit on the floor with your feet together, legs straight, and your body leaning back on your arms and hands. Raise your hips as high as possible, then lower them and relax.

Exercise 5. Lie flat on the floor with your elbows at your sides. Tense the muscles of your back and arms, and then force your hips upward as high as possible. Relax and repeat.

Exercise 6. Raise both legs while lying on floor, keeping your knees straight, and touch the floor with your toes over your head.

Exercise 7. While standing, stretch your arms rigidly in all directions.

Exercise 8. While standing erect, turn your head in all directions.

Exercise 9. Always walk erect. Sit straight and endeavor to be "tall," whether walking, sitting, or lying. In this way you will be conscious of trying to maintain an erect spine.

Each of these exercises should be repeated 10 to 15 times with a short rest after each set.

Group B

Exercise 1. Stand erect, holding a pair of dumbbells at arm's length. Inhale and bend directly sideways. Exhale and return to starting position. Breathe in again and bend to the opposite side. Keep the dumbbells overhead throughout the movement. Bend directly sideways as shown; do not lean forward or backward.

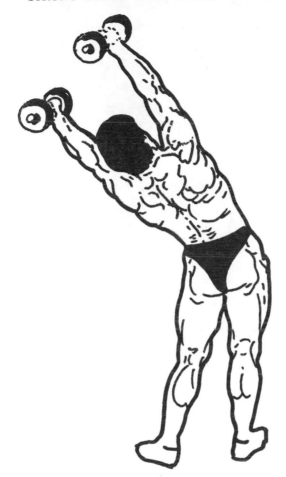

Back Exercise B1

Bend to each side nine times. Add one repetition at every third practice session until you can perform 18 counts correctly, then add 2½ pounds to each bell and start over with nine counts. This exercise will develop the muscles of the side, small of the back, shoulders, and waist.

Exercise 2. Assume the position shown in Fig. 1, placing your feet 24 to 30 inches apart. With a mighty heave and

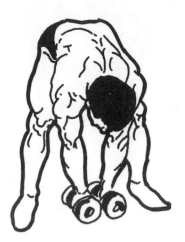

Position 1

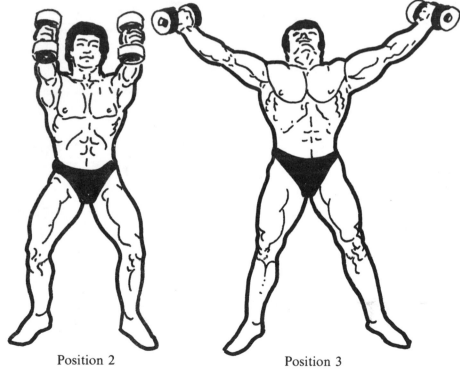

Position 2
Back Exercise B2

Position 3

swing, bring both bells to position 2, breathing in deeply. Your arms should not stop at position 2, but should continue until they are directly overhead, while you continue to inhale deeply. From the overhead position, continue the movement of your arms down and out to position 3. Broaden your chest and shoulders in this final position by bringing your arms backward as far as possible. Return to the starting position while exhaling completely.

Repeat this movement nine times exactly as described, and gradually work up to 18 counts, then add 2½ pounds to each bell and start over with the original count of nine. This exercise is excellent for the entire upper body, front and back, and concealed breathing muscles.

Exercise 3. Bend over from your waist, with your arms hanging straight down toward the floor and gripping dumbbells as shown. Breathing in slowly, raise your arms directly sideways until they are in line with your shoulders. Return your arms to the starting position while slowly breathing out. Keep your back, arms, and legs straight throughout the movement, and do not strain.

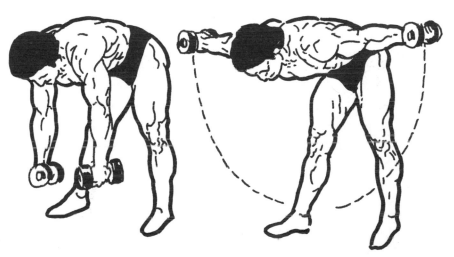

Back Exercise B3

Repeat six times and gradually work up to 12 repetitions, then add 2½ pounds to each bell and start over with the original count of six. Splendid for the lower back muscles, arm triceps, and shoulder muscles.

Exercise 4. To stretch your spine and strengthen your arms and legs, place a bar across your insteps as shown. Draw your knees close to your body, and then begin to push out by straightening your legs. Resist your leg pressure by pulling back with your hands. When this exercise is done properly, your arms, legs, and back will feel the pressure completely. Repeat six to eight times.

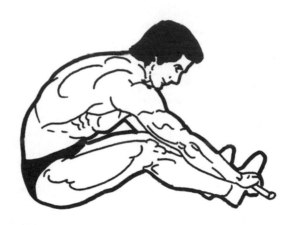

Back Exercise B4

Exercise 5. Stand erect, holding the dumbbells overhead with the palms of your hands facing forward as shown. Simultaneously bend over and bring your arms straight down sideways. When you reach the right-angle position shown, twist the bells around so that your palms are facing the floor. Return to the starting position keeping your arms straight and twisting your hands back to the palms-forward position. Exhale slowly and completely when bending and inhale fully on returning to the starting position. Learn to coordinate the movement, keeping your arms, back, and legs straight throughout. Do not bend beyond a right-angle position. Do not rush through the movement; master it slowly.

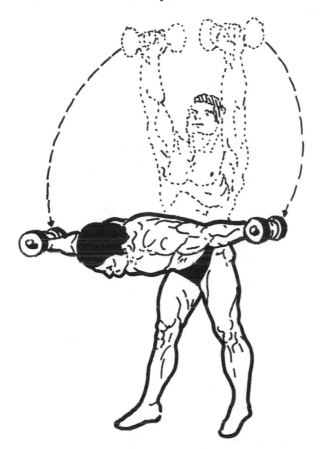

Back Exercise B5

Repeat six times. Add one repetition at every third practice session until 12 counts are made, then increase the weight of each bell by 2½ pounds and start over with six repetitions. This exercise is for upper body development, and also influences the arm and hip musculature from a different angle.

Group C

Exercise 1. Place a barbell on the floor across your feet. Grip the bar with the palms of your hands facing your body as shown. With your back flat and legs straight, simply straighten your back until you are in an erect position. Breathe in as you lift the weight and breathe out as you lower the bar to the floor. Let your back perform this movement; hold the bell with your arms straight.

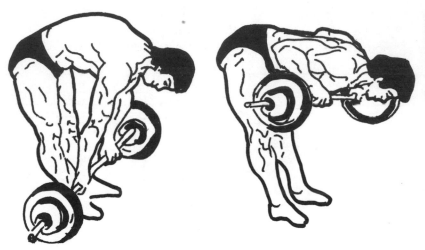

Back Exercise C1   Back Exercise C2

Repeat nine times. Add one repetition at every third practice session until 18 counts are reached, then add ten pounds to the barbell and start over with nine repetitions. For the back, grip, and forearm muscles.

Exercise 2. Keeping your back flat in a right-angle position, extend your arms holding the barbell as in exercise No. 1 of this group. Pull the barbell up to your chest, allowing your arms to travel out from your body. Slowly lower the barbell, extending it almost to the floor. It is not necessary to touch the floor with the bell when lowering it to the starting position. Inhale on raising the bell, exhale on lowering it. Study the illustration carefully. Keep your arms and legs straight and your back flat throughout the movement.

Repeat nine times. Add one repetition at every third practice session until 18 counts are reached, then add ten pounds to the barbell and start over with nine repetitions. Splendid for the lower back, shoulders, and arm muscles.

Exercise 3. Stand perfectly erect, with a barbell resting across the back of your neck, and your hands and feet spaced well apart. Grip the bar with the palms of your hands facing forward. Breathing out, slowly bend your body forward to the right-angle position shown. Allow your hips to move back, and keep your back flat throughout the movement. The upper back muscles that create depth in the back will be most influenced if you hold your head high and keep your elbows tight to your sides.

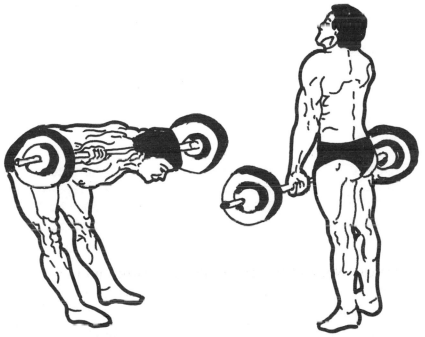

Back Exercise C3   Back Exercise C4

Repeat six times. Add one repetition at every third practice session until you can perform 12 counts, then add ten pounds to the barbell and start over with six repetitions. This exercise is great for the entire back, trims the waist, and stretches the muscles of the hips and the back of the thighs.

Exercise 4. Hold the barbell with your arms extended across your thighs. From this position, raise your shoulders as high as possible toward your ears in a shoulder-shrugging movement. Breathe in as you raise your shoulders and out as you lower them. As you shrug, roll your shoulders around. Stand erect with your feet spaced comfortably apart, holding the barbell with your palms facing your body, keeping your arms straight.

Repeat nine times. Gradually work up to 24 repetitions, then add ten pounds to the barbell and start over with the original count of nine. This exercise aids in developing all of the upper body muscles that influence breadth and depth.

Exercise 5. Stand erect with your feet spaced comfortably apart. Place the barbell across the back of your neck as shown. Breathe in slowly and raise the barbell to arm's length overhead. Breathe out slowly and lower the bell to starting position. Press the weight overhead with pure arm strength.

Repeat six times. Add one repetition at every third practice session until 12 counts are made, then increase the weight of the bell by five pounds and start over from the original count of six. Excellent for the upper back, shoulders, chest, and arm musculature.

Exercise 6. Assume the same position as in exercise 5, spreading your hands and feet well apart. From this position, bend your body from side to side, bending only at the waist. Do not lean forward while bending; incline your upper body slightly backward in order to keep erect. Breathe in and out naturally throughout the movement.

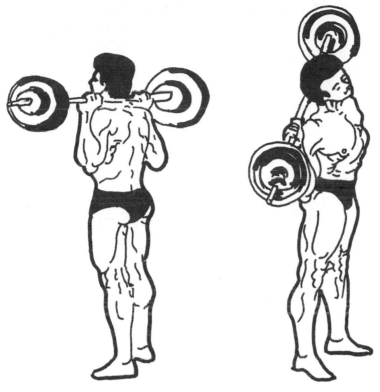

Back Exercise C5   Back Exercise C6

Repeat six times to each side. Add one repetition at every third practice session until you make 12 counts to each side, then add five pounds to the barbell and start over with six repetitions. Great for the side waist muscles and lower back.

Exercise 7. Stand with your feet spaced comfortably apart. Place the barbell on the floor across your feet. Grasp the center of the bar with one hand, palm down, and rest your other hand on your knee. Hold the bell slightly above the floor, letting the weight stretch your shoulder down, then pull the barbell as high as possible with your elbow pointing out as shown. Without pausing, lower the barbell almost to the floor, and repeat. Press hard on your knee with your nonlifting hand. Straighten your legs as you lift the barbell, and keep your back flat. When you have lifted the barbell to the height shown, do not hold it in this position, but immediately breathe out and lower almost to the floor.

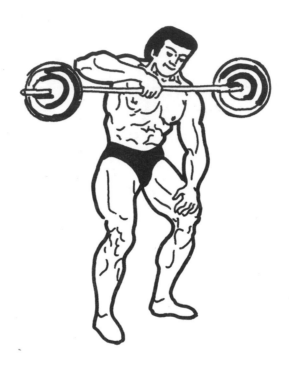

Back Exercise C7

Repeat six times. Add one repetition at every third practice session until 12 counts are made, then add five pounds to the barbell and start over with six repetitions. Perform equally with each arm. Splendid for the arms, back, and legs.

Group D

Exercise 1. Stand erect on a box or stool, holding the barbell across your thighs. Grip the bell with your palms facing your body. Exhale and bend over from the waist, allowing the bell to travel as far past your feet as possible. Return slowly to the erect position while breathing in. Do not attempt this exercise until you have practiced and mastered all of the group A, B, and C exercises. Keep your legs, arms, and back straight. Use only enough weight to master your balance without straining.

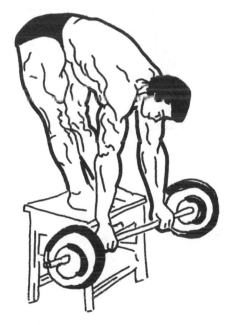

Back Exercise D1

Repeat six times and gradually work up to 12 repetitions, then add ten pounds to the bell and start over with six repetitions.

Exercise 2. Assume the position shown in the illustration. Lift the barbell off the floor and place it behind your neck. Breathe in and raise your body as high as possible. Breathe out and lower your body to the starting position. Breathe in and raise your body as high as possible, this time twisting your shoulders to the right and then to the left as far as possible without straining. Lower and repeat all three movements, always exhaling fully. The table or bench should be fastened to the floor. This movement should not be attempted until you have conditioned yourself with many months of training: harm or injury may result from inadequate conditioning.

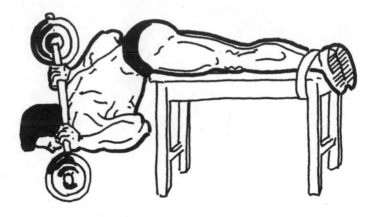

Back Exercise D2

Why You Should Have
a Strong Neck

Many physical educators consider the neck to be a barometer of vitality. A strong, shapely neck is a valuable physical attribute and a sign of bodily vigor.

Apart from the fact that a well-rounded, beautiful neck is the pride of all women, and a well-developed neck imparts an appearance of rugged strength to a man's physique, it also implies great powers of endurance and indicates a great reserve of energy.

Exercising the neck means more than just improving mere muscular appearance. It means the establishment of unrestricted circulation to the brain which is reflected in more buoyant spirits, a happier outlook, and clearer thinking. It helps to soothe away tensions and offers relaxing therapy to the entire head area. Intelligently applied, neck exercises help to eliminate nerve impingement due to faulty alignment of the cervical vertebrae, weak conditions of the throat, and indirectly influence the concealed muscles controlling voice production, perhaps even improving tone and enunciation, besides increasing the ability to talk for long periods without strain.

The benefits of neck exercises should make everyone realize how valuable they are and provide a source of inspiration to practice this vital phase of health and bodybuilding regularly.

There is nothing more unsightly or uncomplimentary than an underdeveloped or overly fat neck. The appearance of the whole upper body is dependent upon the proper symmetry of the neck.

The hollow neck, the protruding Adam's apple, the double chin, the drooping head, and premature signs of wrinkles are but a few of the conspicuous defects directly or indirectly associated with the neck's muscular deficiency.

While you can disguise any undeveloped part of the anatomy with clothing, the neck is one part of the body whose shape and appearance, sooner or later, cannot be successfully covered.

Unfortunately, many people look on their necks only as a convenient or suitable place for draping a collar or some type of fashionable covering. However, the same people are the first to complain when they are suffering with throat soreness, a stiff neck, or any type of neck discomfort that prevents them from functioning properly. Only then do they become aware that they have such a thing as a "neck." However, everyone admires the perfect bodily poise that can be seen throughout the animal kingdom, and the superb carriage and proudly arched necks of the various animals never fail to please the eye.

There is absolutely no excuse for anyone to have a scrawny neck, when a few minutes devoted every day to intelligently applied exercise can change the deficient appearance completely. Overcoming the deficiency and developing a neck of proper size that is well rounded, columnar, and erectly poised on the shoulders is one of the best indications of physical well-being and sturdiness.

The neck serves as a bridge between the brain and the body. The nerve and life impulses originating in the brain must pass through the neck to reach the body. An amazing amount of knowledge can be gleaned by studying the internal and external structures of the neck.

The *cervical vertebrae* (the vertebrae in the neck), are connected to each other by strong ligaments and muscles. In between the muscles run the most important nerves of the body—those which control the action of the heart and respiration. These nerves come directly from the skull, while others branch out from the spinal cord. The blood vessels which service the brain (the *carotid arteries* and *jugular veins*) are also shielded by the muscles of the neck. It is therefore profoundly important that these muscles be kept in good condition. The stronger the neck muscles, the more erect the head is on the shoulders and the better the symmetry of the body; more important, stronger neck muscles condition the vital internal structures.

Other important internal structures—the *trachea, larynx,* and the *esophagus*—are brought under better control, and become healthier, stronger, and less susceptible to colds and disease due to better circulation of the blood brought about by the exercise methods. The blood which nourishes the brain and removes its waste products must pass through the neck. The air on which life depends must pass through the neck on its way to the lungs.

Proper exercise movements will bring about a greater blood supply, and improve function and promote development of all of the neck's correlated structures. The brain and the spinal cord benefit from the development of the neck. Since vitality depends on a good nervous system, you can understand why a strong neck is associated with dynamic vigor and health.

The very life and volatile power of your muscles depends on the nerve supply passing through your neck. The nervous system is largely dependent upon the condition of the neck, for it is here that we find the source of our nervous activity. It continues all the way down the spine, from which it branches out to stimulate the whole body. Everyone who is fortunate enough to be endowed with proper neck structure possesses great concentrated energy. Many exercise enthusiasts fail to realize the importance of developing a columnar neck which can invigorate the whole body and result in improved health and strength.

Neck strength is a wonderful asset. A boxer resisting a

knockout punch will be better off if his neck is strongly formed. Professional wrestlers' necks, although sometimes overdeveloped, have excellent contour and no matter which way their heads are turned or carried, they present a pleasing appearance. Head-to-head balancers also have powerful neck muscles, and their necks are truly remarkable in strength and endurance. I will never forget how impressed I was with the fine carriage and development of the native women in the tropical islands, who balance a heavy basket loaded with their wares on their heads, and walk along as if the load were not even there.

It is not necessary for everyone to develop the huge neck of the athlete or wrestler, but if properly applied exercises are devoted especially to the *trapezius* muscles in the back and also to the *sternocleidomastoid* at the side of the neck, symmetrical lines will shape out the appearance in a very short span of time. A beautiful neck is something to strive for and to be proud of. Exercise as outlined here will make such a possession easily attainable.

The muscles in the neck are many and varied in their purposes. Only a few need be discussed, for these are easily found and their strength tested and, if these muscles are properly exercised, the other neck muscles will become strengthened as a matter of course.

In the front and at the sides of the neck we have the *platysma* muscle. This is a very broad and somewhat thin sheet of muscle which proper exercise of the neck will do much to strengthen and thicken. I will not attempt to give all of the points of origin and insertion of this muscle, as to do so would require a bewildering array of anatomical data. It is enough to say that the upper portion of this muscle is found covering the chin and jaw, and that it extends downward, enveloping the whole front of the neck. The muscle also covers the sides of the neck, and extends down over the collarbone and the shoulder. The action of this muscle causes the wrinkling of the skin on the neck when the neck is brought into extreme muscular action. This muscle serves also to protect the great carotid arteries and the jugular veins.

The various uses of this muscle are too numerous to be given in detail. But it may be said that it draws down the jaw, lowers the underlip, and in many ways affects the expression of the features. Beneath it there is a *fascia,* or sheathing of muscle, that surrounds the neck, and the strength of this fascia (called the deep cervical fascia) is developed by precisely the same work that strengthens and toughens the platysma.

That muscle of the neck which is most readily found, and which is capable of the most visible development, is known as the *sternocleidomastoid.* Found just in back of the lobe of the ear, it crosses the front of the neck obliquely and continues down to the breastbone. In many respects this is the most important muscle of the neck, and it is certainly the most powerful. When the neck muscles are tensed, the sternocleidomastoid should stand out very distinctly. It will feel like a strong, quivering rope to the fingertips.

This muscle originates in two heads; one arises from the upper portion of the breastbone, and the other from the collarbone. At the heads this muscle is separated into its parts, but these gradually merge, and are completely joined at about the middle of the neck. The insertion of this muscle is at the mastoid process behind the ear.

The sternocleidomastoid muscles serve many purposes. When only the muscle on one side of the neck is employed it draws the head over to the shoulder on that side. Another movement of the muscle rotates the head to turn the face to the shoulder on the other side. Its movement is felt very plainly in this motion. If the head is in a fixed position the sternocleidomastoid muscles on both sides are employed together in raising the chest in the act of forced inspiration of breath.

The *trapezius* muscle is located at the sides of the back of the neck and extends out over the shoulders. This is really a muscle of the back, but it will benefit from proper neck work.

Anatomically, the *splenius* muscle is also described as one of the muscles of the back, but it plays so important a part in the work of the neck that I will say a few words about it here. The splenius may be felt in the tensed neck just in back of the sternocleidomastoid. It runs obliquely up and forward, beginning in the upper portion of the back and ending in the neck.

The splenius is a broad, flat muscle of considerable toughness. As it ascends into the neck it divides into two portions, one of which is known as the *splenius capitis* and the other as the *splenius cervicis.* The capitis is inserted mainly at the mastoid process, and the cervicis into the two or three upper vertebrae of the neck. These splenius muscles are employed in drawing the head directly backward; they also aid in drawing the head to one side, and somewhat in rotating it. The most important function of the splenius muscle is to keep the head in an erect position.

When exercising the neck, extra care should be taken not to apply the resistance too vigorously at the start, because overstraining the muscles will produce a kink or stiff neck. These are very discouraging and unpleasant, and the pain may last for several days. Begin all neck movements slowly. Take it easy, and coax your neck rather than force it. Remember, your objective is to train, not to strain, and that you are interested in physical construction as opposed to physical destruction.

You will note that there are four groups of neck exercises. Practice each group in sequence. Start with group A. Do not advance until you have practiced all of the movements within a group and perfected your performance. In this way, you will develop the muscles properly and avoid strains and discomfort.

Neck Exercises

Group A

Exercise 1. Stand erect. Without moving any part of your back or shoulders, turn your head to the right. Turn it back again, carrying it past the face-forwards position until it is turned to the left. Repeat the full movement from side to side four to six times.

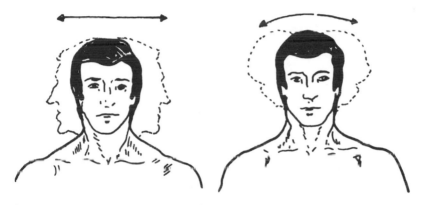

Neck Exercise A1   Neck Exercise A2

Exercise 2. Stand erect. Without moving your back or shoulders, bend your head over to the right. Bring it back again past the upright position until it is bent over to the left. Repeat the movement from side to side four to six times.

Exercise 3. Stand erect. Without moving your back or shoulders, bend your head forward. Bring it back again past the upright position until it is bent backward. Repeat the movement from front to back and back to front four to six times.

Exercise 4. Stand erect. Without moving your shoulders or back, rotate your head on your neck, beginning the rotation to the right and making as big a circle as possible.

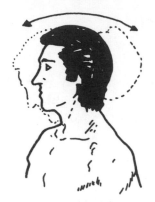
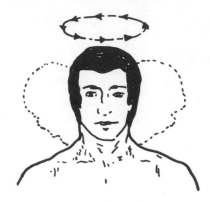

Neck Exercise A3   Neck Exercise A4

Repeat in this direction a number of times, and then reverse the rotation so that it begins to the left. Repeat again a number of times. Do not continue the movement long enough for any giddiness to occur, even though there may be no strain or feeling of discomfort in the muscles.

Coordinating movements of the neck

The blending of the two movements, as described in exercises 5 and 6, will help to prevent tension, discomfort, stiffness, and restriction of the weak musculature.

Exercise 5. Stand erect. Without moving any part of your back or shoulders, continue a turning movement of your head from left to right as in exercise 1 of this group of neck movements, and at the same time bring your head first forward, and from this position past the upright position, until it is carried fully backward, as in exercise 3. From there, bring your neck forward again and so on.

Exercise 6. Stand erect. Without moving any part of your back or shoulders, continue a bending movement of your head from left to right as in exercise 2 of this group of movements, and at the same time carry your head forwards and backwards as in the previous movement.

These movements are invaluable to those who are

predisposed to neck weaknesses. At the beginning, restrictions in the parts brought into play may cause some difficulty in carrying out the movements. However, it is these very restrictions which have to be overcome, and the movements will do this naturally and easily if they are carried out with restraint and within the control of the upper neck joint and the chest, back, and neck muscles. Under no circumstances should any attempt be made to force the action of the joint. Each exercise will bring greater ease until all the movements can be carried out with ease and freedom within the range of the motion.

Group B: Movements of the lower neck joint linking the neck with the body

The joint which is brought into play in these movements is the one which connects the neck with the body. The head should not incline or the neck bend as they are carried out. Both head and neck should move as one column on the shoulders, with any bending of the neck reduced to a minimum.

Exercise 1. Stand erect. Without moving any part of your back or shoulders, and without inclining your head either to the right or left, or forward or backward, thrust your neck forward. Bring your neck back past the upright position until it is thrust fully backward. Repeat four to six times.

Exercise 2. Stand erect. Without moving any part of your back or shoulders and without inclining your head, move your neck to the right. Bring it back past the upright position until it is carried fully to the left. Repeat four to six times.

Exercise 3. Stand erect. Without moving any part of your back or shoulders and without inclining your head, rotate your neck, beginning the rotation to the right and making as big a circle as possible. Repeat a number of times and then reverse the rotation, beginning it to the left. Repeat a number of times.

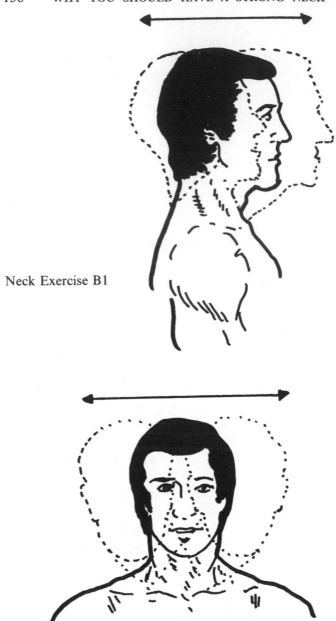

Neck Exercise B1

Neck Exercise B2

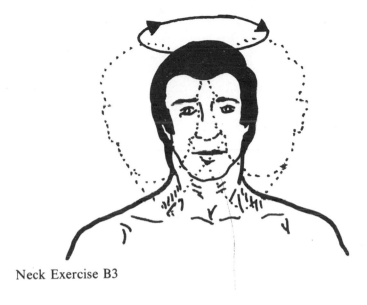

Neck Exercise B3

Group C

Exercise 1. Stand or sit perfectly erect with your fingers interlaced as shown in the illustration, grasping the back

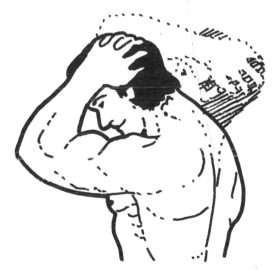

Neck Exercise C1

of your head. Pull your head forward to your chest, at the same time resisting with your neck. Return your head backward, resisting with your hands. Learn to use your arm resistance with gradual control, smoothly and without the slightest jerk.

Practice this exercise nine times, and very gradually increase the number of counts to 18. Develops the muscles at the back of the neck.

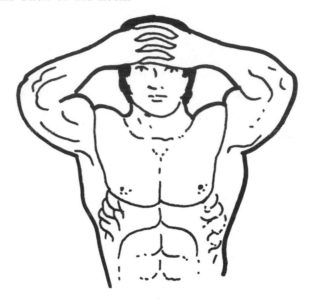

Neck Exercise C2

Exercise 2. With the palms of your hands, fingers interlaced and pressed against your forehead, force your head forward and downward against your hands. Then reverse the movement, pushing your head backward against the resistance of your throat muscles. This movement is especially recommended for those who have a flabby or wrinkled condition of the front of the neck. It can be made more effective by drawing down the corners of the neck during the exercise.

Practice nine times, and gradually increase the number of counts to 18. This exercise develops the muscles of the throat and the front of the neck.

Exercise 3. Place your right hand against the right side of your head. Push your head toward your left shoulder, resisting with your neck. Return your head toward your right shoulder against the resisting pressure of your right hand.

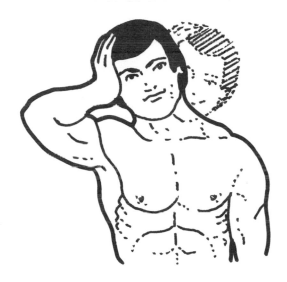

Neck Exercise C3

Practice this exercise nine times for the right side of your neck. Repeat for the left side. Gradually increase the number of counts to 18 in both directions. Develops the muscles at the sides and front of the neck.

Exercise 4. Stand or sit erect and roll your head completely round and round by bending your neck in a circular motion, moving first in one direction and then in the opposite direction. This exercise makes the muscles and joints of the neck flexible and free moving (not illustrated).

Advanced Neck Exercises

Group D

As an advanced form of neck exercise, you can begin to use the headstrap for neck development. Many valuable exercises can be performed with this apparatus.

When using the headstrap, do not bend over too far. Maintain a well-balanced position to avoid neck kinks. Use your hands on your thighs as a source of control. This will help prevent body motion, as all movement must be performed with your head and neck only.

Further advanced exercise consists of lifting heavier weights. When you can perform all of the group D movements 16 times, increase the weight slightly. For best results, perform these exercises three or four times a week. Aim to perfect your performance at all times. Each exercise must be performed smoothly and without bodily motion. The weight employed must always be within your control.

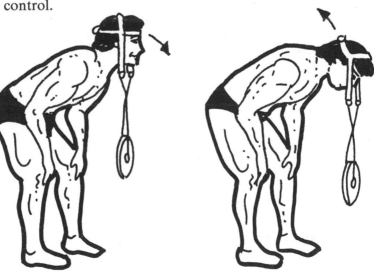

Neck Exercise D1

Exercise 1. Lift your head backward and forward from chest to shoulder, as shown in the illustration.

Exercise 2. Move your head from side to side.

Exercise 3. Follow through with the movements performed in exercises 1 and 2, rotating your head in a complete circular motion.

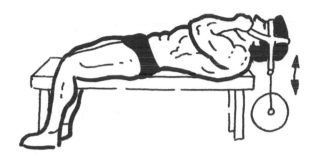

Neck Exercise D4

Exercise 4. Lie on your back on a bench or bed with your head extended over the edge as illustrated. From this position, raise and lower your head as far as possible. Next, lie on your stomach and perform the movement to the same extent. Then lie on your side, and exercise both sides of your neck equally.

Exercise 5. Rest your head and neck on a cushion or folded blanket. From position 1, slowly and steadily push upward until you are in the complete bridge position (position 2). Steadily return to position 1. Do not jerk your body up or pry onto your head by forcing back with your legs. Confine the movement and effort to your neck muscles. During the back and forth movement, keep your feet braced and help to push with your legs no more than is necessary to perform the complete movement.

Progress slowly. Start with nine repetitions and gradually work up to 18 counts.

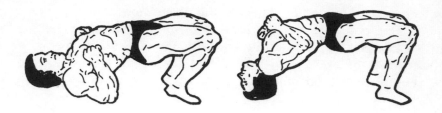

Position 1   Position 2
Neck Exercise D5

Exercise 6. This exercise is the reverse of exercise 5. Face down, with your body supported on your forehead, and your hands and feet assisting your balance. Slowly push forward slightly with some hand assistance until your head assumes the position shown in the illustration. From this position, work your head slowly backward, forward, and from side to side until tired.

This exercise is excellent for the development of the muscles on the front of the neck, as well as those on the side of the neck, and for filling out any hollows over the collarbones.

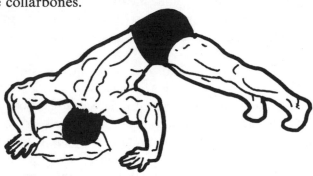

Neck Exercise D6

You, Too,
Can Build Strong Arms

Throughout the pages of literature the deeds of men with strong arms have been freely glorified. The romance attached to these members of the human anatomy has almost no equal. They were the prime agents employed in defending the weak, protecting innocence, and vanquishing the unworthy. Even Longfellow raised his voice in praise of them, for who does not recall these familiar lines from the *Village Blacksmith*?

> *And the muscles of his brawny arms*
> *Are strong as iron bands.*

From boyhood on, most men are impressed by well-developed arms, and there are few who don't envy them. Some men find pride in developing their arms to great size and strength. I confess that from my early school days I longed to have arms that would compare with those of the hard-working smith, as pictured by the poet, and at a comparatively early age I set about acquiring them.

Years ago, quite by chance, I came across a health publication which illustrated the arms of various strong men and the exercises they had used in their development. Most of the exercises were executed with various apparatus, including chest weights, barbells, and heavy dumbbells.

Not having funds to purchase such equipment at the time, I practiced a few of the exercises illustrated without any apparatus. It wasn't entirely satisfactory but it gave me the clue I needed. I saw that I had to use my body in a manner that would furnish the necessary resistance to serve as a substitute for the apparatus.

This led to my investigation of various systems of exercise, and before long, my research completed, I put it into practice. Soon I could see the good results of my method, for the value I received from those exercises was entirely beyond estimate.

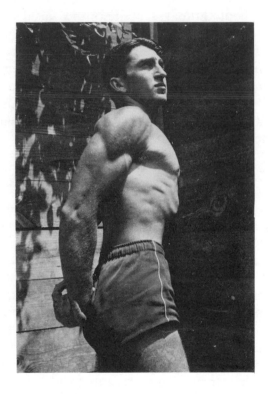

Vic Boff at 19 years of age. Note the powerful arm and shoulder development.

The purpose of this chapter is to show you how I developed powerful arms and how you can also acquire them in a fairly easy manner. When your arm muscles are balanced in development, your increased strength will be astounding. In practically no time, if you are persistent and intelligent in the application of your exercises, you will be able to handle your own body weight with absolute ease, and lift weights you never dreamed of being capable of lifting.

Naturally you need to develop other parts of the body along with your arms, but a good part of that will come as a matter of course in doing all that will be outlined for your arm development. So proceed with the following exercises, and see if your wishes are not realized before long.

Briefly, there are four muscles in the upper arm, 22 in the forearm, and 18 in the hand. Suffice it to say, the *biceps* muscle on the front of the arm bends the arm at the elbow. In other words, it flexes the arm by bringing the forearm and upper arm closer together and takes on a ball-like appearance. This is the muscle that is employed in pulling, tugging, or lifting anything, or in hauling.

Now, in order to straighten the arm, the *triceps* muscle lying on the back of the upper arm is called into play. Its work is to straighten out the arm after the biceps have flexed it. This muscle acts contrary to the biceps. The triceps are the arm's powerful extensors. They give the arm a beautiful rounded appearance when fully developed.

It is important not to develop one muscle at the expense of the other. No matter how large your biceps becomes, if it lacks the relative triceps development, the physical ability and shape of your arm will be inferior to the man who has a smaller arm with a better-balanced appearance. In fact, it would be anomalous for a man to possess splendidly developed biceps and relatively weak triceps.

Arm Exercises

Group A
Triceps exercises

Exercise 1. The floor dip is an exercise which will develop the triceps along with the muscles of the back, chest, and shoulders. Lie on the floor, facing down, supporting your body on your hands and toes. Keep your body perfectly rigid and lower it slowly by bending your arms until your chest touches the floor. Then raise your body, and continue until tired. When you have mastered 20 movements correctly, continue with the following exercises.

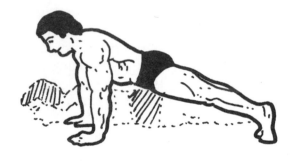

Arm Exercise A1

Do not hold your breath in this type of movement, or in any of the arm-dipping movements. Exhale going down, and inhale slowly while pressing back to starting position.

Exercise 2. Place two chairs facing each other about 24 inches apart. Put the palm of each hand on the seat of a chair. Extend your feet along the floor until your legs are straight, and at the same time keep your body rigid. The position of your body is the same as in exercise 1. From this position, bend your arms and lower your body slowly as far as possible between the chairs.

Keep your elbows tight to your sides, and without raising your hips or changing the position of your body, press yourself back to arm's length. Repeat slowly until tired. The farther apart the chairs are, the greater the effect on the chest muscles. The farther in front of the hands and shoulders the chairs are, the greater the effect on the front shoulder muscles. Exercise equally in both of these positions, and aim for balance.

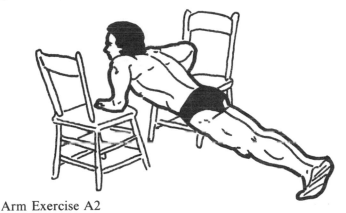

Arm Exercise A2

Exercise 3. This exercise uses the same arrangement as in exercise 2, but with the body in a reversed position. That is, instead of face downward, it will be face upward, with the body resting on the heels instead of the toes. The palms of the hands will be resting on the seats of the chairs with the fingers pointing backward. This is important. Now, lower your body slowly between the chairs as far as you can go. Then rise, straightening your arms. Do not heave your body in order to help the movement. Continue until tired.

Exercise 4. The following triceps builder is more advanced in nature and requires more exertion than the previous exercises. Place two chairs back to back about 20 inches apart, so that there is enough space between them for you to stand with a hand grasping the back of each chair. Now raise your feet off the floor, slowly lowering your body as far as possible. Then slowly press your body back to the straight-arm position—without swinging your body.

Gradually increase this type of dipping until you can perform it 30 or more times consecutively. Remember that your objective is to cultivate and train, but not to strain or tear yourself down. Other advanced exercises that are particularly effective for the triceps are handstanding, Roman ring work as performed by a gymnast, wrestling, and rowing. Overhead lifting with barbells and dumbbells is also good.

Biceps Exercises

Exercise 5. Stand erect with your arms at your side. Now place your left hand in your right palm, still keeping your right arm directly at your side. While holding your left hand, bend your right hand toward the wrist. Next, begin to bend your right arm at the elbow, resisting vigorously with your left hand. Continue until your hand is brought to your right shoulder. This movement brings the right-arm biceps forcibly into play as it overcomes the left-arm pressure.

Bring your arm back to the original position, but in doing so, resist the downward motion by pulling up with your left hand. In performing this exercise, reverse your hands in order to develop both arms equally. What you put into it is what you will get out of it (not illustrated).

Exercise 6. Chinning the bar is also a great biceps developer. Grip the bar with the palms of your hands facing you, and with your arms perfectly straight. Now draw your body up using the strength of your arms until your chest touches the bar. In this manner, you get complete biceps action. Hold the position for a second,

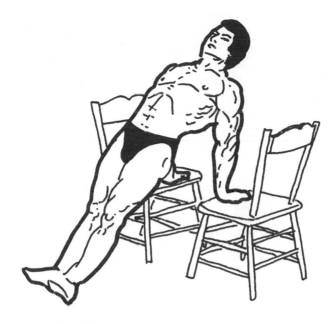

Arm Exercise A3

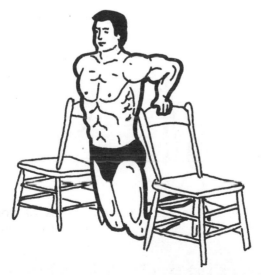

Arm Exercise A4

then slowly return to the starting position. Continue slowly until tired.

A variation of this is to grip the bar with your hands reversed—that is, with the backs of your hands facing you this time. When you become fairly proficient, make the exercise more difficult by gripping the bar with only one hand and assisting the movement by holding your wrist with your other hand. Remember to use both arms; aim for symmetry.

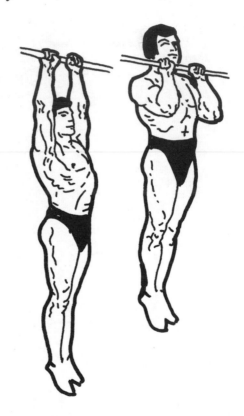

Arm Exercise A6

Other work and exercise which can be very beneficial for biceps development are rope climbing, wresting, wrist turning, and above all, the exercise known as the two-handed slow curl with a barbell or dumbbells. This is the same as exercise 5; the only difference is that it is performed with weights.

Forearm Exercises

Exercise 7. To develop your forearms, take a newspaper and grasp one end with one hand, holding it at arm's length in front of you. Try to roll the paper into a ball by slowly manipulating it with your fingers. Do not cheat—try to accomplish this work solely with your fingers. You will find that this is an excellent finger, wrist, and forearm developer. You can also take magazines and newspapers, double them up, and try to tear them in half. This is fine work for the same muscles.

Exercise 8. The wrist roller is a tremendous exercising appliance for the forearms, wrists, and gripping muscles. Bore a hole through the center of a wooden roller. Run a strong, four-foot cord through the hole, tying several knots in one end to prevent slipping. On the other end of the cord, attach a small weight or dumbbell—three to six pounds to start. Gradually add more weight.

Assume an erect position, with your arms extended directly in front, palms down. Roll the rope around the stick until it is wound completely around the roller. Then

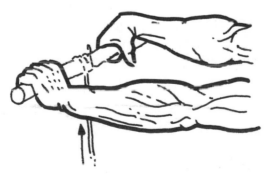

Arm Exercise A8

reverse your hands and assume a palms-up position and repeat. Wind in each position two or three times.

Learn various movements which will give a twisting and turning action to the arms. Dip on your fingers instead of your palms, and try to do away with one finger at a time. This type of exercise will give your forearms and wrists ample work to develop that vise-like grip.

Dumbbell Exercises

Group B

Exercise 1. Stand erect, with your arms straight at your sides. Hold the dumbbells with the palms of your hands facing forward. Very slowly bend your forearms upward to your shoulders. Inhale slowly on the upward movement and exhale on extending your arms back to the starting position. Keep your upper arms stationary. Do not grip the sides of your body with your upper arms or allow your elbows to rest on your body. The more you turn your thumbs away from your body as you are curling the bells, the greater the resistance placed on your biceps muscles.

Repeat nine times. Add one repetition at every third practice session until 18 counts are performed, then add 2½ pounds to each bell and start over with nine counts. Excellent for the upper arm muscles, especially the biceps.

Exercise 2. Stand erect, keeping your arms tight to your sides, and your palms up with the thumbs turned out. Bend forward slightly. Keep your arms straight and raise them backward as far as possible. When your arms are extended to the limit, twist your hands to the right and then to the left as far as you can. Note the dotted line in the illustration. Slowly return to starting position. Be sure to keep your arms straight and tight to your side and your palms facing forward.

Repeat six times. Add one repetition at every third practice session until you can perform 12 repetitions easily, then add 2½ pounds to each bell and start over with six counts. Excellent for the upper arms, especially for the triceps muscles on the back of the arm.

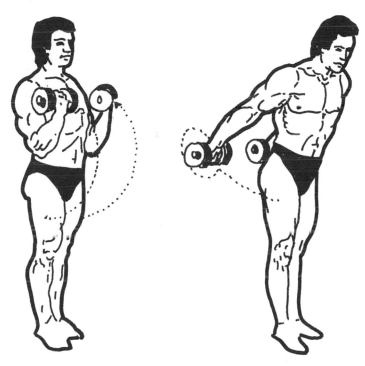

Arm Exercise B1   Arm Exercise B2

Exercise 3. Stand erect with your arms held straight out in front at shoulder level. Grip the bells with your palms facing down, as in position 1. Breathe in and allow your arms to travel outward and sideways until they are in line level with your shoulders. Twist your palms upward and then flex your upper arms at the elbows. Tense your hands for a few seconds, as in position 2. Return to starting position while breathing out. Cultivate good style in this movement. Keep your arms straight before flexing, keeping your elbows high and on a level with your shoulders. Twist your hands and tense your arm muscles when flexing for greater effect. Study the illustrations carefully before attempting this exercise.

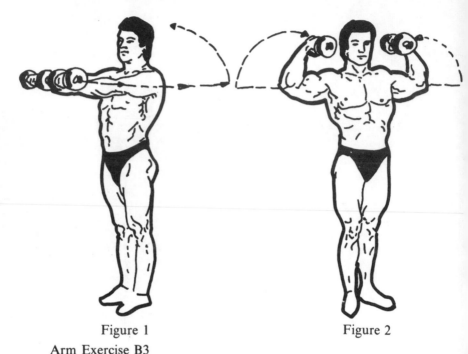

Figure 1   Figure 2

Arm Exercise B3

Repeat six times. Gradually work up to 12 perfect repetitions and then add 2½ pounds to each bell and start over with six repetitions.

Exercise 4. Assume the same position as in exercise 1, with the exception that the palms of your hands must face down while gripping the dumbbells. Very slowly bend your forearms upward to your shoulders. Bend your hands down on the wrists, so as to get plenty of forearm action as

you curl the bells to your shoulders. Inhale on raising the
bells and exhale on returning to the starting position. Use
only your arms to perform the movement, and put plenty
of grip and effort into it.

Repeat eight times. Add one repetition at every third
practice session until 16 are performed, then add 2½
pounds to each bell and start over with eight repetitions.
Great for the forearm and biceps.

Exercise 5. Assume the same position as in exercise 1.
Begin to curl or flex your arms with the palms of your
hands facing down. As you flex your arms, turn your
hands and wrists, bringing the fronts of your hands toward
your shoulders as shown by the dotted line in the
illustration. As your hands return to the starting position,
turn your hands and wrists again so that your palms face

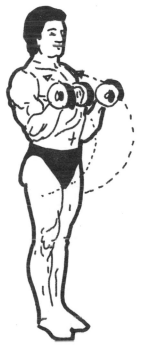

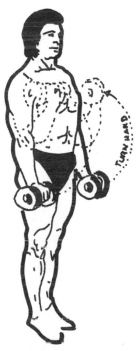

Arm Exercise B4   Arm Exercise B5

down. This movement can be reversed for diversification. That is, instead of beginning with your palms facing down and ending with your palms facing up, you can begin palms up and end the curl palms down. Study this movement carefully before beginning.

Repeat eight times. Add one repetition at every third practice session until 16 are performed, then add 2½ pounds to each bell and start over with eight repetitions. It's great for the forearm and biceps and for the triceps and wrist muscles involved as well. This exercise will prevent knotty muscles; the biceps is being extended as it is contracting.

Exercise 6. Stand erect, holding the barbell at a right angle to your body as shown by the dotted line in the

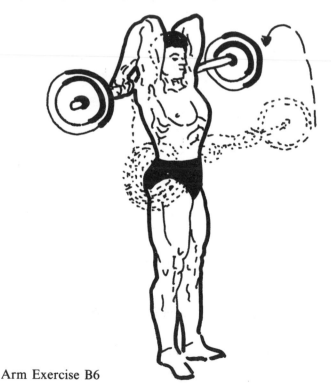

Arm Exercise B6

illustration. From this position, curl the barbell to the back of your head as shown. Breathe in as you curl and exhale as you return to the starting position. Grip the bar with your palms up and hands shoulder width apart. Keep your elbows pointed forward in this movement.

Practice six times. Add one repetition at every third practice session until 12 are performed, then add five pounds to the barbell and start over with six repetitions. Splendid for the arms, shoulders, lower chest, and back.

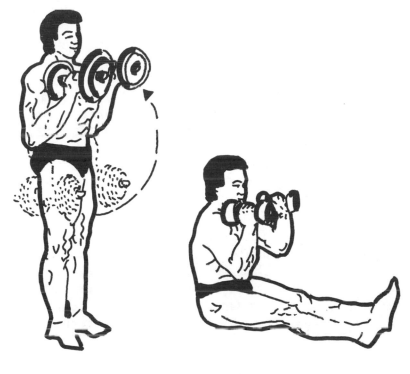

Arm Exercise B7   Arm Exercise B8

Exercise 7. Stand erect, holding the dumbbells fully extended at your sides as shown by the dotted lines. Curl the dumbbells to your shoulders exactly as shown. Breathe in as you curl and out as you lower the dumbbells to your sides. Keep your posture erect. Do not allow your elbows to move backward or to grip your sides. For variation, make this exercise work the shoulder and triceps. When the bells reach shoulder level, follow through by pressing them to arm's length overhead. Repeat in exactly the same manner as stated.

Repeat nine times. Add one repetition at every third practice session until 18 are performed, then add five pounds to each bell and start over with nine repetitions. Great for the upper arms and forearm muscles.

Exercise 8. Assume a sitting position as shown, with the bells held at shoulder height. Slowly raise the bells to arm's length overhead, looking up as you complete the movement. Keep your heels on the floor, and keep your back straight. Breathe in all the way as you extend your arms, and breathe out as you lower the bells to your shoulders. For perfect performance, extend your arms fully overhead and do not let your heels leave the floor.

Repeat six times. Add one repetition at every third practice session until 12 are performed, then add five pounds to each bell and start over with the original count of six. For arm, shoulder, back, and chest muscles.

Exercise 9. Assume the position shown in the illustration, with one dumbbell held at your side. Grip the bell with your palm facing forward. From this position, extend your arm backward as far as possible. Resist the movement by pressing hard with your free hand on your knee, bending forward as shown. Breathe in as you extend your arm backward, and breathe out as your arm returns to the starting position. Do not allow your body to bend further forward than shown. Keep your lifting arm straight and close to your side, and do not twist your body.

Repeat six times. Add one repetition at every third practice session until 12 are performed, then add five pounds to the bell and start over with the original count of six. Excellent for the triceps muscles on the back of your arm.

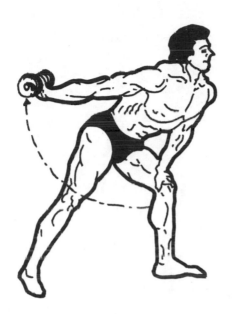

Arm Exercise B9

Exercise 10. Stand perfectly erect with the dumbbells held at your sides as shown in the illustration. Slowly curl the bells under your armpits as shown. Breathe in as you flex your arms and out as you lower the bells to the starting position. Hold your chest high and your head back. Keep your elbows pointed out in a straight line with your shoulders as you lift your arms under.

Repeat six times. Add one repetition at every third practice session until 12 are performed, then add five pounds to each bell and start over with the original count of six. Works the biceps, forearms, and wrist muscles from a different angle to influence perfect development.

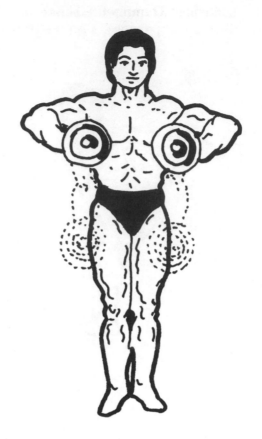

Arm Exercise B10

Important points to observe

Study the illustrations and text carefully. Learn to perform each exercise correctly and with good form. Remember to balance your arm-training program. Select a few triceps exercises along with a few biceps movements. Aim for perfection in your workouts, and you will be rewarded with a strong and symmetrical pair of arms. Those individuals who cannot master the dipping exercises should start with the dumbbell training program.

Barbell/Dumbbell Routine

Group C

These exercises are excellent triceps and shoulder developers. Repeat each exercise six times and gradually work up to 12 repetitions.

Exercise 1. The military press. Lift a barbell to your shoulders and then stand perfectly erect. Keeping your knees braced and your trunk erect, steadily press the barbell to arm's length overhead. Lower to the starting position and repeat. Inhale while pressing the barbell overhead and exhale as the bar is lowered.

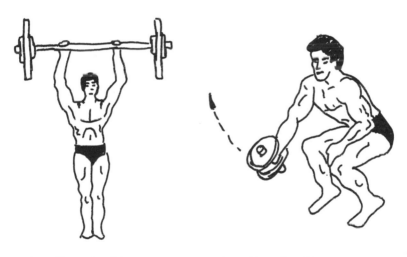

Arm Exercise C1   Arm Exercise C2

Exercise 2. One-hand swing as an exercise. Stand erect, with your feet about 15 inches apart, placing a dumbbell on the floor between your feet, handle facing forward. Keeping your back straight, bend your knees and grasp the bell with your right hand, placing your left hand on your left knee. Keeping your lifting arm straight, swing the bell forward and upward to about shoulder level, assisting the movement by pressing down with your left hand. Allow the dumbbell to swing back between your legs, and repeat the movement, but this time swing the dumbbell to full arm's length overhead while either splitting or dipping your legs. Repeat with your other arm.

Exercise 3. The alternate press. Lift a pair of dumbbells to your shoulders and stand erect. Maintaining an upright position, press the right dumbbell to arm's length overhead. Lower the right dumbbell back to your shoulder, simultaneously pressing the left bell to arm's length overhead. Breathe freely and naturally throughout.

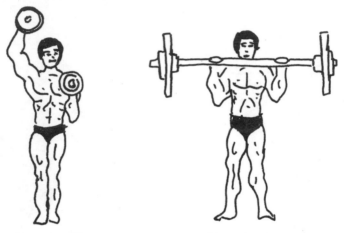

Arm Exercise C3   Arm Exercise C4

Exercise 4. Press behind neck. Lift a barbell to your shoulders, then lift it over your head and lower it to a "behind the neck" position. Keeping your trunk erect and knees braced, steadily press the barbell to arm's length overhead. Lower back behind your neck and repeat. Inhale as the press is made, and exhale as the bar is lowered.

Exercise 5. Press on back (on bench). Lie back on a bench or form, holding a barbell in your hands at your shoulders. Steadily press the barbell to arm's length above your chest, simultaneously inhaling deeply. Lower the barbell to your chest and repeat.

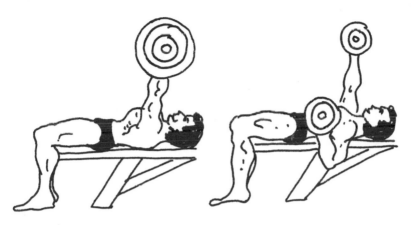

Arm Exercise C5   Arm Exercise C6

Exercise 6. Press on back on bench with dumbbells. It is performed exactly like the preceding exercise, using dumbbells. Alternate arms in pressing to arm's length overhead.

Put Some Stretch into Your Muscle-Building Program

Take a tip from the most muscular, most powerfully dynamic animals in the world, the mighty jungle cats—tigers, lions, leopards, cheetahs—and put stretching exercises into your training routine. The only regular exercise any jungle cat ever takes, apart from the demands of everyday living, is stretching. The big cats do a lot of stretching after sleeping or resting for any length of time. Their "claw-sharpening" against tree trunks is really a form of stretching. It involves plenty of reaching, pulling, tensing, and relaxing.

These jungle cats stretch naturally, instinctively, to improve muscle tone, to increase their flexibility, to build more muscles and strength, and to improve circulation. All wild animals do some stretching—it is normal, natural, and beneficial. Only man has lost the art of stretching and this is partly responsible for his rapid physical deterioration.

Stretching is probably the most natural form of exercise. It is an exercise which is practiced instinctively after a period of inactivity; for example, after sleep or when the body has been held too long in a cramped position. It is nature's way of telling you to awake from your muscular idleness or to relieve abnormal pressure on the blood vessels and nerves.

Stretching exercises are not developing movements.

166

They are freeing movements—relieving any part of the body from discomfort, restriction, or stiffness. The moment you expand, extend, or "reach out" any part of your body when nature asks, you are relieving undue tension.

Although stretching movements are lacking in all the various movements a muscle can perform, they are the only type of activity that allows for a strong contraction of certain muscles followed by a complete relaxation.

When the extensor muscles are extended and contracted to their fullest extent, the flexor group are relaxed. This allows the muscles to be kept at their normal length.

Freeness of the body joints—being flexible and supple, having an erect carriage—shows that we are youthful, while the opposite conditions are signs of old age.

Since stretching is nature's way of reminding us of our muscular idleness, we can extend that instinctive response into a few minutes of conscious stretching and obtain more of the constitutional benefits it offers.

There are many ways in which a system of stretching can be devised. You can use your body naturally without any apparatus and stretch your limbs to their fullest extent while standing, sitting, and reclining. Or you can hang from a horizontal bar with your body fully extended, with one or both hands gripping the bar, and perform various stretching movements. You can also stretch your chest and arm muscles by extending your arms across a doorway and letting your body sway forward. However, you must be very careful not to strain from overstretching or overreaching. Each movement should be carried to its fullest extent. Relax when beginning your exercises and impart that amount of vigor to the movement that is within your bodily strength.

There are hundreds of different kinds of stretching exercises and it is a good idea to do a few of these when you get up in the morning, a few more during the day, and still more just before you go to bed at night. In fact, whenever you feel the urge to stretch—go to it, because this is nature's way of telling you that your muscles, blood vessels, nerves, or other vital organs need some stretching exercise.

Simple Stretching Exercises

Group A

Exercise 1. Stand erect with your legs apart. Raise your arms high above your head with your fingers extended. At the same time, rise up on your toes and try to touch the ceiling. Repeat a number of times. Vary this by raising your toes off the floor.

Exercise 2. Stand erect with your hands clasped behind your head. Turn your entire trunk to the right as far as it will go. Then turn your trunk to the left as far as it will go. Repeat a number of times.

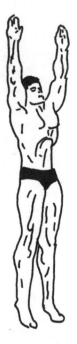

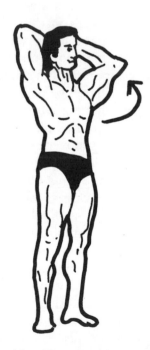

Stretching Exercise A1   Stretching Exercise A2

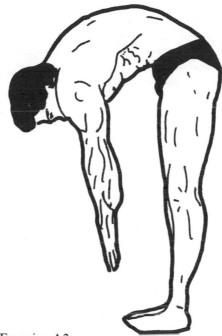

Stretching Exercise A3

Exercise 3. Stand erect with your feet apart, and bend your trunk forward, then backward, then to the right, and then to the left. Repeat a number of times.

Exercise 4. Sit on the floor with your legs extended and spread apart. Place your hands on the floor in front of you and try to touch your chest to the floor by sliding your hands forward. Repeat a number of times.

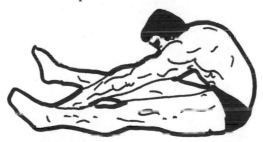

Stretching Exercise A4

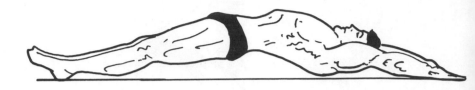

Stretching Exercise A5

Exercise 5. Lie flat on your back with your arms stretched out beyond your head. Point your toes and keep stretching your entire body until your back comes off the floor. Stretch with all your might and then relax your body. Repeat a number of times.

Advanced Stretching Exercises

Group B

Exercise 1. Place the heel of one foot on the back rest of a kitchen chair. Keeping both legs straight, lean forward and wrap both arms around your outstretched leg. Press down hard. Then stand erect again and stretch both arms overhead. Repeat a number of times. Perform the same exercise with your other heel on the chair.

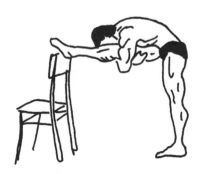

Stretching Exercise B1

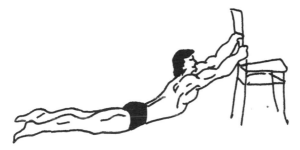

Stretching Exercise B2

Exercise 2. Lie face down facing the back legs of a chair. Reach forward with both hands and grasp these legs. Gradually climb up the chair legs with your hands so that your back gets a good stretch, as shown in the illustration. Climb down with your hands to the starting position. Repeat a number of times.

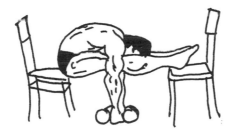

Stretching Exercise B3

Exercise 3. Place two chairs facing each other. Sit on the edge of one chair and place your heels on the edge of the other. Grasp a dumbbell in each hand and raise these overhead. Now bend forward, allowing the dumbbells to pass to the outside of your legs, and keep bending forward until your chest is resting on your knees and the dumbbells are as close to the floor as they will go. Straighten your trunk up again and raise both arms overhead to the starting position. Repeat a number of times.

Keep Your Feet
Healthy and Happy

Foot health is of major importance in our daily lives. Our health and general physical efficiency depends on our feet to an appreciable extent. Physical endurance, the vital factor in bodily efficiency, is largely controlled by feet that can withstand the terrific daily pressure they must bear.

The human foot is subjected to more physical discomforts than any other part of the body. Not only do the feet have to bear the natural burden of body weight and carry on the function of locomotion, but in many cases they also have to withstand the abuses of faulty footwear, long hours of continual standing when certain occupations require it, the shock of walking on unnatural pavements, and the weakness that obesity brings because of the increase in body weight without a corresponding increase in the strength of the foot muscles. To top it all, mechanical deficiencies of the body such as poor posture, improper walking techniques, etc., add to the daily wear and tear on the feet.

Briefly, the foot is composed of 26 bones and a network of ligaments, nerves, tendons and muscles, veins and arteries. The *sciatic* nerve, which is the largest nerve in the body, has its terminal branches in the nerves of the foot. The entire structure is so correlated that the slightest undue pressure or disturbance sets up an irritated nerve condition of pain. Continued neglect of the feet can lead to other impaired bodily conditions.

Keeping the feet in good condition depends on wearing shoes that are properly designed and correctly fitted. Shoes which are narrow with pointed toes are the cause of many foot troubles, as are high-heeled shoes. The former type of shoe gives rise to painful corns and callouses and hinders the balance of foot muscles. The high-heeled shoe throws the whole body out of balance and interferes with the muscles on the bottom of the foot.

Since shoes are a vital necessity for everyday living, you should wear shoes that give your feet sufficient room to expand when weight is put on them, with soles broad enough to support your feet in every part and a low and broad heel, made of leather which is flexible enough to permit play of the muscles. Shoes should be changed frequently to rest the feet and also for better hygiene. When not in use, shoes should be kept in shoetrees to hold their shape. It is also important to wear socks which are large enough to give your feet and toes full freedom of movement.

Bathing your feet for a few moments in cold water after exercising them is advantageous. This will further strengthen and refresh them. A foot bath of cold and hot water, changing quickly from one to the other, is also fine for the feet. A brisk rubbing with a dry, rough towel is also beneficial.

Since human feet were not designed to be encased in shoes, you should exercise them "bare" as often as possible. The exercises which follow must never be performed while you are wearing shoes, since full action of the muscles must be secured. Never strain your feet while exercising them. Your object should always be to condition and train them for perfect foot health.

Natural Foot Exercises

Exercise 1. Raise your heels up off the floor as high as possible. Lower and repeat until your arches are slightly tired.

Exercise 2. Raise your toes up as far as possible. Lower and repeat about 40 times.

Exercise 3. Pick up marbles with your toes, and try to throw them with your feet. The more clawlike and arched you make your feet, the more you will develop the muscles that hold up your arches.

Exercise 4. Walk with short strides, with your toes in and heels out. Cross your feet, keeping your toes in, and attempt to grasp with them.

Exercise 5. Bend your toes down as far as they will go, until you can feel a pull on the muscles of your leg. Repeat 25 to 50 times.

Exercise 6. Stand with your feet parallel, and raise the inner borders. Repeat 25 to 50 times.

Exercise 7. Walk barefoot—especially on sand or grass —as much as you can.

Exercise 8. Keep your feet parallel when walking, with your toes pointing straight ahead and your weight on the outer edges of your feet. Walk at least one to two miles a day.

Exercise 9. At times when you are sitting down, cross your feet and rest them on their outer edges. This permits better relaxation and circulation.

Know Your Muscles

While it is not necessary for you to study the anatomy of the body thoroughly, it would be to your advantage to learn the names, locations and actions of the muscles of your body. You will find their names and locations in the following charts.

Examine yourself periodically before a mirror. If your inspection indicates that some part of your body is not responding to training as you desire, you can select exercises designed to develop these particular muscles.

The location and general form of the external muscles of the body are illustrated in the following drawings, showing the front, back and side of the Farnese Hercules, made in 1721 by M. B. Gucht, a sculptor and anatomist of that day. Although the drawings show a body that is developed beyond the norm, they provide a visual conception of the sources of man's power.

NOTE: In *Physical Culture* magazine, October, 1930, David P. Willoughby, an American writer and investigator in the field of physical development, assembled the supplemental data upon the action and methods of developing these muscles that accompany the Farnese Hercules drawings.

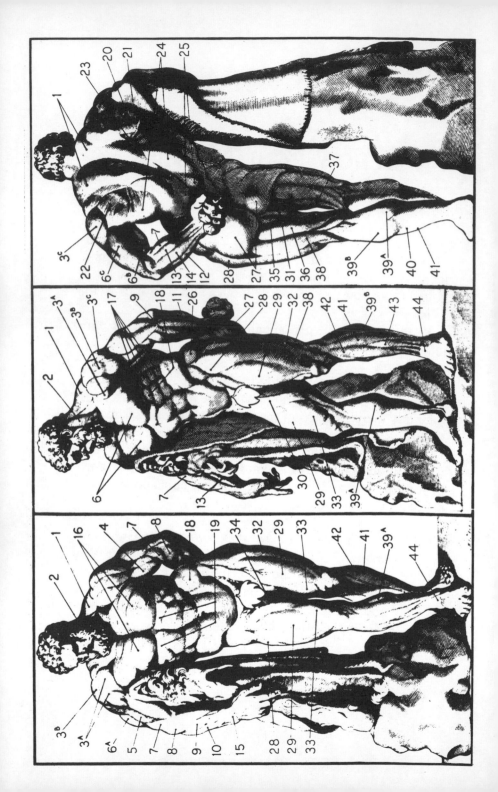

SUPERFICIAL MUSCLES IN MAN

NO.   LATIN NAME AND MEANING

1. Trapezius (Table-shaped).
2. Sternocleidomastoid (From attachments of muscle).
3. Deltoid. A—Anterior. B—Lateral. C—Posterior. (From Greek letter Delta, meaning triangular).
4. Biceps Brachii (Two-headed flexor of forearm).
5. Brachialis (Front muscle of arm).
6. Triceps Brachii (Three-headed extensor of forearm). A—Outer Head. B—Inner Head. C—Long Head.
7. Brachioradialis (Arm muscle).
8. Extensor Carpi Radialis Longus (Long extensor of radial side of wrist).
9. Extensor Carpi Radialis Brevis (Short extensor of radial side of wrist).
10. Extensor Digitorum Communis (Common extensor of digits).
11. Extensor Carpi Ulnaris (Extensor of ulnar side of wrist).

12. Flexor Carpi Ulnaris (Flexor of ulnar side of wrist).
13. Flexor Carpi Radialis (Flexor of radial side of wrist).
14. Palmaris Longus (Long palmar muscle).
15. Posterior Annular Ligament of Wrist.
16. Pectoralis Major (Breast muscle).
17. Serratus Anterior (Saw-toothed muscle).
18. Obliquus Externus Abdominis (External muscle of abdomen).
19. Rectus Abdominis (Straight muscle of the abdomen).
20. Teres Minor (Smaller round muscle).
21. Teres Major (Greater round muscle).
22. Infraspinatus (Muscle below the spine).
23. Rhomboideus Major (Larger rhomb-shaped muscle).
24. Latissimus Dorsi (Broadest of the back).
25. Lumbar Aponeurosis (Tendon of loins).
26. Gluteus Medius (Middle buttock-muscle).
27. Gluteus Maximus (Largest buttock-muscle).

28. Tensor Fasciae Latae (Tightener of the broad fascia).
29. Rectus Femoris (Muscle of thigh).
30. Sartorius (Tailor's muscle).
31. Gracilis (Slender muscle).
32. Vastus Lateralis (Immense outer muscle).
33. Vastus Medialis (Immense inner muscle).
34. Adductor Longus (Long adductor).
35. Adductor Magnus (Great adductor).
36. Semitendinosus (Half-tendon muscle).
37. Semimembranosus (Half-membrane muscle).
38. Biceps Femoris (Two-headed flexor of the leg).
39. Gastrocnemius (Leg muscle). A—Inner Head. B—Outer Head.
40. Soleus (Sole-fish muscle).
41. Peroneus Longus (Long fibular muscle).
42. Tibialis Anterior (Anterior tibial muscle).
43. Extensor Digitorum Longus (Long extensor of the digits).
44. Anterior Annular Ligament.

FUNCTION	ACTION IN WEIGHT-LIFTING	OTHER ACTIVITIES
1. Draws head backward and to one side.	Overhead lifts.	Wrestling. Hand-balancing. Roman ring work.
2. Draws head forward; rotates head; assists in lifting chest.	Influenced by lifts involving the trapezius muscle.	Wrestling. Head-balancing. Boxing.
3. Raises arm to horizontal.	Overhead lifts. Arm lifts to horizontal.	Hand-standing. Balancing. Wrestling.
4. Flexes and supinates forearm; flexes and adducts arm.	Lifts to shoulders—Repetition lifts.	Chinning. Rope-climbing. Roman ring work. Wrestling.
5. Flexes forearm.	Same as No. 4.	Same as No. 4.
6. Extends forearm. Draws arm back.	Overhead lifting; "pressing" or "jerking."	Hand-standing. Dipping. Roman rings. Wrestling.
7. Flexes forearm and assists in supination.	Same as for No. 4.	Same as for No. 4.
8. Extends hand; with flexor abducts hand.	Lifting barbell to shoulders.	Bending spikes and iron bars.
9. Extends hand.	Same as for No. 8.	Same as for No. 8.
10. Extends fingers.	As in No. 8.	Piano-playing; spaced-typing, etc.
11. Extends hand; with flexor carpi ulnaris adducts hand.	All lifts to the shoulder or overhead.	Bending bars. Card-tearing. Floor-dipping on finger-tips. One-finger lifts.
12. Flexes and adducts hands.	Same as for No. 11.	Similar as for No. 11.
13. Flexes and pronates hand; abducts hand.	Same as for No. 11.	Same as for No. 11.
14. Tightens fascia of palm, and then flexes hand.	Same as for No. 11.	Similar to No. 11.
15. Holds bones and tendons of wrist.		
16. Draws arm inward and forward. Rotates arm inward.	Lifts performed while lying on back.	Dipping. Chinning. Rope-climbing. Roman ring work. Wrestling.
17. Draws shoulder forward. Other uses.	Similar to No. 16.	Similar to No. 16. Boxing, fencing, throwing.
18. Compresses abdomen; rotates pelvis.	One-hand lifts, "bent press," and side presses.	Tumbling. One-hand lifts with another person.
19. Flexes body; depresses thorax; compresses abdomen.	All one- and two-hand overhead lifts where trunk is bent backward.	Tumbling. Wrestling. Jumping. Rowing. Leg-raising.
20. Rotates humerus.	Overhead lifts.	Ring-work. Wrestling.
21. Draws down and rotates arm inward.	Lying lifts.	Chinning. Rope-climbing. Rowing.
22. Rotates humerus.	Same as for No. 20.	Same as for No. 20.
23. Draws scapula up and inward.	Similar to No. 21.	Similar to No. 21.
24. Draws arm down and rotates it.	Similar to No. 21.	Similar to No. 21.
25. A thin, tendinous covering joining lower back muscles.		
26. Abducts thigh; rotates it inward.	Lifts developing thigh and hip extensors.	Ballet Dancing. Wrestling. Tumbling.
27. Extends thigh, and rotates it outward.	"Quick" lifts. Back and harness lifts.	Sprinting. Jumping. Hill-climbing. Wrestling.
28. Tightens fascia latæ.	Same as for No. 26.	Same as for No. 26.
29. Extends leg; flexes thigh.	All "quick" lifts. One- and two-hand dead lifts. Back and harness lifts.	Sprinting. Cycling. Jumping. Tumbling. Hill-climbing. Wrestling.
30. Flexes thigh and leg; rotates leg inward and thigh outward.	Lifts developing thigh and hip extensors.	Ballet and acrobatic dancing. Jumping. Wrestling. Tumbling.

31. Adducts thigh and leg; flexes leg.	Influenced by lifts which develop thigh and hip.	Same as No. 34.
32. Extends leg.	All "quick" lifts. Back and harness lifts.	Cycling. Sprinting. Jumping. Tumbling. Wrestling. Hill-climbing.
33. Extends leg.	Same as for No. 32.	Same as for No. 32.
34. Adducts, rotates outward, and flexes thigh.	Influenced by lifts which develop thigh and hip extensors.	Ballet and acrobatic dancing. Wrestling. Horseback riding.
35. Adducts thigh.	Same as for No. 34.	Same as for No. 34.
36. Flexes leg and rotates it inward; extends thigh.	Two-hand (and one-hand) dead lift. All "quick" lifts.	Same as for No. 27.
37. Flexes leg and rotates it; extends thigh.	Same as for No. 36.	Same as for No. 36.
38. Flexes leg and rotates it; extends thigh.	Same as for No. 36.	Same as for No. 36.
39. Extends foot; flexes leg.	Dead-weight lifting.	Sprinting. Cycling. Walking. Jumping. Wrestling.
40. Extends foot and rotates it inward.	Similar to No. 39.	Similar to No. 39.
41. Extends, abducts and everts foot.	Similar to No. 39.	Similar to No. 39.
42. Flexes foot and elevates inner border.	All "quick" lifts of flat-footed "squat."	Similar to No. 39.
43. Extends the four small toes.	Involved as in No. 39. and 42.	Involved as in No. 39.
44. Holds bones and tendons of ankle in place.		

Food, Diet, and
the Health Builder

The role of food and diet in building a strong, healthy, and beautiful body is certainly one of the most important questions in the life of every health builder.

I have often heard people say, "What is so important about nutrition, as long as you eat three square meals each day?" They fail to realize that it isn't a question of eating enough of *any* kind of food, but rather of eating the *right* kind of food, properly prepared.

It also is a shame that many of our athletes know very little about diet. As a result, we occasionally find them suffering from boils, pimples, colds, and whatnot.

Food is our most profound everyday habit, but many of us do not consider it important enough to try to understand it. However, the food we eat determines not only our strength and energy, but even the question of whether or not we are going to be sick or well.

There weren't any refined foods generations ago, and as a result the hardy person of that era automatically obtained a diet rich in all the valuable vitamins and minerals his body needed. There was little need for nutritional education.

Today, our foods are often refined. It is estimated that about 66 percent of all calories eaten come from foods which have had most of the vitamins and minerals removed. Transportation, storage, drying, and canning cause a further loss of food value which did not occur years ago when each family had its own garden. Therefore, left to chance, our choice of foods can rarely produce health. It follows that your nutrition must be planned.

In simple terms, the purpose of food is two-fold. It must nourish the body, and it must maintain it in good health. With this fundamental duality firmly in mind, we can solve the problem of balancing our diet without losing our way in a jungle of technical terms.

The true purpose of scientific research is to discover natural laws or principles and how they work. The laws governing nutrition are simple and easily understood.

It is an established principle that Nature balances each of her foods to play their part in healthy nutrition. Whole foods make an all-round contribution to the body's nourishment and its efficiency. It is only when we process them in such a way as to disturb the balance and relationship of their component food elements that they fail to do their job effectively.

There are seven component elements of food—proteins, carbohydrates, fats, vitamins, minerals, roughage, and water. These food elements may be divided into two classes.

The first three—proteins, carbohydrates, and fats—are nutritive. They make up the bulk of what we eat, and provide most of the body's substance. The remaining four elements—vitamins, minerals, roughage, and water—are chiefly concerned with maintaining and protecting the health of the body.

The health-giving food elements are essential. They make it possible for the body to digest and use the nutritive elements. Their presence in sufficient amounts means that the food we eat can be used to the full and metabolized into living flesh and blood, pulsating with health and vigor. They also allow the proper neutralization and elimination of residual wastes and toxins produced by the body.

The sum and substance of all the discoveries in food

science narrows down to this: the way to a healthful balanced diet is to base it on the foods which are balanced in themselves. The narrower the range of foods, the more essential it is to choose balanced whole foods that make a contribution to the health as well as the nourishment of our bodies.

Generally speaking, there are two ways of eating. You can eat to fill your stomach and temporarily appease hunger and appetite. Almost any food will do this. Or you can eat balanced natural foods, chosen with the object of satisfying the complete nutritional needs of your body. There is no reason why the second way should not be just as enjoyable as the first, with the added advantage that the real hungers of the blood and body cells for first-class building and servicing materials will be satisfied, as well as the hunger of the stomach.

When the diet is properly balanced to meet the needs of the body for protein, carbohydrates, minerals, and vitamins, perfect performance in building and repair will be taking place throughout its billions of cells, producing needed energy. Each organ will carry on its work normally, and when all the waste products are adequately removed, superb health and vitality will become a reality.

The average person is in danger of not getting ample qualities of the essentials for normal nutrition because of deficiencies in foods themselves, and because the average family's conception of diet is still dominated by traditions and empirical notions. Over a period of time this can be harmful because nutritional imbalance induces deficient body conditions. This can mean poor muscle tone, pallor and rough skin, undue muscle and joint pains, constipation, and many other ills and complaints.

The maintenance of optimum nutritional intake and balance should be the guiding principle of all food planning. The following descriptions of the various types of food will give you an idea of how to select them for your diet.

Proteins

Proteins are utilized to build, maintain, and repair the nerves, muscles, blood, bones, skin, and all other tissues of the body. They are made up of molecules or building blocks called amino acids. The body needs 22 different amino acids to maintain its structure. It can synthesize 14 of these from foods, but eight of them must be supplied intact and are known as the "essential" amino acids. The proteins in foods differ in the number and variety of amino acids they supply. Therefore, it is usual to draw a distinction between foods supplying essential amino acids, calling them first-class protein foods, and foods which only supply some of the essential amino acids.

First-class or complete protein foods are chiefly of animal origin. They include lean meat, liver and other organ meat, fish, eggs, milk, cheese, and fowl. Nuts, peas, beans (especially soybeans), and whole cereals are also rich in protein. All natural foods provide some proteins, but the amount in most of them is comparatively small.

An excellent variety of protein-rich supplements or concentrates made from meat, fish, milk, or soy powder can be obtained from most health food stores.

The average man and woman should have about one gram of complete protein daily to every two pounds of *normal* weight (not overweight).

Carbohydrates

Carbohydrates are the chief energy-producing nutrients. They serve as bodily fuel, and yield energy in the form of heat and muscular power; they can also be transformed and stored as fat in the body. They are divided into two groups—foods which provide carbohydrates in the form of starch, and foods which provide them in the form of sugar. The starch-rich foods include breads, potatoes, cereals, spaghetti, beans, dried corn, rice, etc.

The "B" vitamins are found in whole, unrefined, unde-
natured food, and for this reason, it is wisest to eat most of
your starchy foods in their natural state. For similar
reasons, the natural sugars are to be preferred to the pure,
refined, white variety which is entirely vitaminless and
mineral-less, and can only do harm when eaten in excess.
Unsulfurated molasses, uncooked honey, ripe bananas,
and dried unsulfurated fruits such as figs, dates, raisins,
apricots, prunes, pears, apples, etc., are excellent natural
sources.

The amount of carbohydrate food eaten should be
related to bodily activity. An active man needs more
carbohydrates than a sedentary one. When restrictions
must be made in the diet, it is the foods in this group that
can be most readily spared. If more carbohydrates are
eaten than the body can use at once, the excess is stored in
the tissues as fat.

Remember to strictly avoid foods made of white flour
and white sugar: cakes, cookies, pies, breads, jams, jellies,
candies, soft drinks, etc. These refined carbohydrates bring
absolutely nothing to the diet except empty calories.

Fats

Although fats have the most calories, their chief nutrient
purpose is to provide slow-burning fuel for keeping the
body warm, lubricated, and organically efficient.

Fats are found principally in whole milk, cream, butter,
egg yolk, cheese, nut butters, vegetable oils, etc. The best
sources of fats are the cold pressed natural vegetable oils
such as safflower, sunflower, soybean, or corn oil, all of
which contain essential unsaturated fatty acids. Avoid the
hard or saturated fats, trim fat from meats, and avoid fried
foods and gravies.

Eat fats moderately and discriminately, for excess leads
to digestive difficulties and when too much fat is combined
with high-carbohydrate meals, a potential weight problem
will become a reality.

Health-Protective Foods

With the protein, carbohydrate, and fat content of
the diet assured, you must make provision for the health-
protective foods. It should be emphasized that the more
active you are, the greater your need for vitamins, food-
minerals, regulating roughage, and water will be. Major
food items that may be classified as health-protective are
all fresh fruits and leafy vegetables in season, natural
seeds, and whole grains with the germ still intact. In any
sport or bodybuilding, it is important that the increased
intake of nutrient foods not push health-protective foods
out of the diet. You will not accomplish anything by eating
extra food if this leads to the omission of fruit or salads in
the meal.

Good nutrition lies in eating foods containing both
nutrients and health-protective foods in proportions
planned to the body's needs according to the demands
made on it.

The vital vitamins

Although so much has been written about vitamins in
recent years, it is still astonishing how many people,
seemingly well fed, suffer from health that is below par
because they do not eat enough of the foods containing
them. Vitamins do more for vitality and vigor than any
other food element.

In fact, there could be no life—human, animal, or
plant—without vitamins. They are the chemical messen-
gers which help provide heat and energy from the foods
we assimilate, promote growth, and repair and rebuild
body cells and tissue. They are the vital link in the chain
that converts crude nutriments in your body into the
tissues that make up your skin, bones, eyes, hair, and
teeth.

You cannot be vital, keen of mind, and have buoyant
health without an ample daily supply of vitamins.

Many factors make it difficult to satisfy our daily needs for all the nutritional, vitamin, and mineral essentials. Loss of potency in both vitamins and minerals occurs due to transportation, storage, processing, and improper methods of preparing food for the table. Faulty eating habits and food fads are other causes of inadequate nutrition.

There is no doubt that lack of vitamins in our daily diet upsets the delicate machinery of the body and leads to nutritional disturbances and disease. Therefore it is most important that our daily menu be consistent in its use of natural foods; foods that millers, bakers, and cooks have no opportunity to damage.

The vitamins are essential to the growth and development of the body. In addition, each vitamin possesses certain important characteristics with which everyone should be familiar.

Study the charts that follow, and you will begin to understand the natural sources of vitamins and minerals, their special roles (functions), and the results of vitamin deficiencies. A working knowledge of the functions of vitamins and minerals should become a part of everyone's matter-of-fact health information.

If you have a nutritional or other specific problem that you find difficult to overcome, you should seek the help of a physician who is an expert on nutrition.

However, when there are restrictions on the diet or when adequate nutrition cannot be obtained from natural foods, natural vitamin-mineral preparations and supplements (powders, tablets, and capsules), made from natural sources, are available. This type of food supplement insures a wonderful supply of concentrated, dynamic nutrition to meet the body's needs for building and energy metabolism. These unique nutritive products are equally good for those who have balanced diets—but you should remember that these preparations are to be used only as a supplement to the very best diet you can obtain.

The food minerals

Minerals are just as important to life as the indispensable vitamins, although we hear less about them. They are vital raw materials of bodybuilding, entering into the formation of bones, sinews, and muscle tissues. They are needed for the healthy functioning of every organ. Calcium is needed by the heart and bones. Iron is as indispensable to the skin as it is to the blood. Phosphorus works with calcium in forming supple cells, and it is also essential to the brain and nerves.

We know less about the other minerals, but it is apparent that iodine, magnesium, copper, zinc, and fluorine all have significant roles in maintaining the harmony of health. Basically, minerals come from the soil in which food crops are grown, so the answer to the problem of getting enough minerals in our food is simply a matter of eating vegetables, fruits, and whole grains in good variety. Minerals also appear in animal foods—milk, cheese, eggs, meat, etc.—nurtured on mineral-rich plant fare, and in the food products of the sea.

Water

Most foods are bulky with moisture, and the water in foods is the best for internal regulation and for making up the body's secretions and excretions. The amount you need to drink in liquid form will vary with the weather but it will also be affected by the amount you get in food. We need from 1½ to 2 quarts of liquid daily, but the more we get in moist foods—fruits and vegetables—the better for health.

Roughage

Finally, there is roughage, the indigestible fiber of food which ensures the regular and efficient elimination of waste food residues from the bowels. Here again, the key is to include adequate whole, unrefined foods plus some fruits or vegetables in each meal.

Planning for Good Nutrition

The essence of good nutrition is to choose some foods from each of the nutrient groups set out here, add a variety of health-protective foods, and the essential needs of your body will be met. The more active you are, the more you need of all foods to maintain your superior well-being.

In the selection of a healthful and strength-building diet it is not enough to ensure that the tissue-building or protein foods and the fuel food elements are present in sufficient quantities, and that they balance each other in a proportion corresponding to your bodily requirements. It is also important to consider the quality and character of these foods. Therefore, avoid what are known as deficient foods, foods that are robbed of their minerals and vitamins—in other words, their natural goodness. This means white flour, white bread, white sugar, pastries, syrups, or any foods that contain considerable amounts of white flour or white sugar. Instead of these deficient foods use whole grain flour, whole wheat bread, and raw sugar or honey for sweetening purposes. Avoid foods which have gone through many processes.

It is very important to eat a raw salad and fresh ripe fruit every day. This will provide your body with the alkaline protective elements (minerals and vitamins) it needs. Avoid too many mixtures and kinds of food at a meal. An excellent plan is to eat one meal consisting of a protein or two, little or no starch, salad or steamed vegetables, and fresh fruit. Vary this with another meal consisting mostly of a starch or two, steamed vegetables, and a sweet dessert. If you suffer from digestive disturbances, this plan will help you to overcome them. You can vary your breakfasts with eggs, whole grain cereals, sweet fruits, etc.

See that your vegetables are cooked in as little water as possible, without soda and condiments. Vegetables which are boiled in lots of water with soda lose most of their health-giving natural salts. Use fats wisely. All forms of fat are better uncooked. Good butter with as little salt as possible, cold pressed olive oil and nut oil, and fresh cream are excellent. Cooking in fat tends to make food more difficult to digest (this means fried foods), but oil or butter can be added to cooked vegetables when served.

Excessive seasoning with salt, sugar, spices, and condiments should be avoided; use them sparingly or not at all. You should also avoid tea and coffee as much as possible.

Shopping for health

Learning to shop for health is an art. The large health food stores stock a wide, almost complete variety of health and organically grown foods. Here you can purchase all kinds of whole grain foods and flours, dried fruits, fresh organically grown fruits and vegetables, dairy and meat products, cold pressed unhydrogenated vegetable oils and nut butters, and protein supplements and natural vitamins as necessary for dietary supplementation.

Artificial coloring, flavor, preservatives, and additives in foods are not to be tolerated. The pure food law protects you somewhat. *Read your food label.* You should make it your business to find out whether any of the changes and processes to which foods are subjected before they reach you have impaired their nutritional worth and vital qualities. Foods that are so changed should be rejected. When we tamper with nature's products, we do so at our own peril. No form of life can be supported wholly on laboratory products; man is no exception to this fundamental law.

Eat nothing at all unless you are entirely comfortable in mind and body. Overeating is the worst dietary error. Food taken in excess of the body's actual needs is worse than wasted. It becomes toxic to the body, and it overtaxes the organs of digestion since nature provides only enough digestive juices to handle the body's needs. A paramount rule which you should observe at all times is to eat slowly and to chew your food thoroughly.

Vitamin-Mineral Chart—Current Usage

Note: The symptoms noted in these pages could occur only when the daily intake of the vitamins mentioned has been less than the minimum daily requirement over a prolonged period. These nonspecific symptoms alone do not prove a nutritional deficiency but may be caused by a great number of conditions, or have functional causes. If these symptoms persist, they may indicate a condition other than a vitamin or mineral deficiency.

Vitamin A

Also known as the Anti-Infective or Anti-Ophthalmic Vitamin. Usually measured in U.S.P. Units.
Natural Sources: Colored fruits and vegetables, dairy products, eggs, margarine, fish liver oils, liver.
Functions: Builds resistance to infections, especially of the respiratory tract. Helps maintain a healthy condition of the outer layers of many tissues and organs. Promotes growth and vitality. Permits formation of visual purple in the eye, counteracting night blindness and weak eyesight. Promotes healthy skin. Essential for pregnancy and lactation.
Deficiency: May result in night blindness, increased susceptibility to infections, dry and scaly skin, lack of appetite and vigor, defective teeth and gums, retarded growth.

Vitamin B-1

Thiamine, Thiamine Chloride. Also known as the Anti-Neuritic or Anti-Beriberi Vitamin. Generally expressed in Milligrams (mgm.), occasionally in Units. 333 Units of B-1 equal only 1.0 mgm.

Natural Sources: Dried yeast, rice husks, whole wheat, oatmeal, peanuts, pork, most vegetables, milk.

Functions: Promotes growth, aids growth and digestion, essential for normal functioning of nerve tissues, muscles and heart, necessary for proper metabolism of carbohydrates and fats.

Deficiency: May lead to loss of appetite, weakness and lassitude, nervous irritability, insomnia, loss of weight, vague aches and pains, mental depression and constipation. In children, a deficiency may cause impaired growth.

Vitamin B-2

Riboflavin or Vitamin G. Measured in Milligrams (mgm.).

Natural Sources: Liver, kidney, milk, yeast, cheese, and most B-1 sources.

Functions: Improves growth, essential for healthy eyes, skin and mouth, promotes general health.

Deficiency: May result in itching and burning of the eyes, cracking of the corners of the lips, inflammation of the mouth, bloodshot eyes, purplish tongue.

Vitamin B-6

Pyridoxine. Measured in Milligrams (mgm.). If it is designated in Micrograms (mcgm.) remember that it requires 1000 Micrograms to equal 1.0 Milligram (mgm.).

Natural Sources: Meat, fish, wheat germ, egg yolk, cantaloupe, cabbage, milk, yeast.

Functions: Aids in food assimilation and in protein and fat metabolism; prevents various nervous and skin disorders; prevents nausea.

Deficiency: May result in nervousness, insomnia, skin eruptions, loss of muscular control.

Vitamin B-12

Commonly known as the "red vitamin." Cobalomin. Since it is so effective in small dosages, it is the only common vitamin generally expressed in Micrograms (mcgm.).
Natural Sources: Liver, beef, pork, eggs, milk, cheese.
Functions: Helps in the formation and regeneration of red blood cells, thus helping to prevent anemia; promotes growth and increased appetite in children; a general tonic for adults.
Deficiency: May lead to nutritional and pernicious anemias, poor appetite and growth failure in children, tiredness.

Vitamin C

Ascorbic Acid, Cevitamic Acid. Expressed in Milligrams (mgm.), occasionally in Units. 1.0 mgm. equals 20 Units.
Natural Sources: Citrus fruits, berries, greens, cabbages, peppers. (Easily destroyed by cooking.)
Functions: Necessary for healthy teeth, gums and bones; strengthens all connective tissue; promotes wound healing; helps promote capillary integrity and prevention of permeability; a very important factor in maintaining sound health and vigor.
Deficiency: May lead to soft gums, tooth decay, loss of appetite, muscular weakness, skin hemorrhages, capillary weakness, anemia.

Vitamin D

Viosterol, Ergosterol, "Sunshine Vitamin." Measured in U.S.P. Units.
Natural Sources: Fish liver oils, fat, eggs, milk, butter, sunshine.

Functions: Regulates the use of calcium and phosphorus in the body and is therefore necessary for the proper formation of teeth and bones. Very important in infancy and childhood.

Deficiency: May lead to rickets, tooth decay, retarded growth, lack of vigor, muscular weakness.

Vitamin E

Tocopherol. Available in several different forms. Formerly measured by weight (mgm.)—now generally designated according to its biological activity in International Units (I.U.).

Natural Sources: Wheat-germ oil, whole wheat, green leaves, vegetable oils, meat, eggs, whole grain cereals, margarine.

Functions: Exact function in humans is not yet known. Medical articles have been published on its value in helping to prevent sterility; in the treatment of threatened abortion; in muscular dystrophy; prevention of calcium deposits in blood vessel walls. Has been used favorably by some doctors in treatment of heart conditions. Much further research needs to be completed before a clear picture of this vitamin will be obtained.

Deficiency: May lead to increased fragility of red blood cells. In experimental animals deficiencies led to loss of reproductive powers and muscular disorders.

Vitamin K

Menadione.

Natural Sources: Alfalfa and other green plants, soybean oil, egg yolks.

Functions: Essential for the production of prothrombin (a substance which aids the blood in clotting); important to liver function.

Deficiency: Hemorrhages resulting from prolonged blood-clotting time.

Nicotinic Acid (Niacin)
Niacinamide (Nicotinamide)

The functions and deficiency symptoms of these members of the B Complex are similar. Niacinamide is more generally used since it minimizes the burning, flushing and itching of the skin that frequently occurs with Nicotinic Acid.
Natural Sources: Liver, lean meat, whole wheat products, yeast, green vegetables, beans.
Functions: Important for the proper functioning of nervous system. Prevents pellagra. Promotes growth. Maintains normal function of the gastrointestinal tract. Necessary for metabolism of sugar. Maintains normal skin conditions.
Deficiency: May result in pellagra, the symptoms of which include inflammation of the skin, tongue; also gastrointestinal disturbance, nervous system dysfunction, headaches, fatigue, mental depression, vague aches and pains, irritability, loss of appetite, neuritis, loss of weight, insomnia, general weakness.

Calcium Pantothenate

Pantothenic Acid. A member of the B Complex family.
Natural Sources: Liver, kidney, yeast, wheat, bran, peas, crude molasses.
Functions: Not yet clearly defined. Helps in the building of body cells and maintaining normal skin, growth, and development of central nervous system. Required for synthesis of antibodies. Necessary for normal digestive processes. Originally believed to be a factor in restoring gray hair to original color, but this function has not been substantiated.
Deficiency: May lead to skin abnormalities, retarded growth, painful and burning feet, dizzy spells, digestive disturbances.

Folic Acid

A member of the Vitamin B Complex.
Natural Sources: Deep green leafy vegetables, liver, kidney, yeast.
Functions: Essential to the formation of red blood cells by its action on the bone marrow. Aids in protein metabolism and contributes to normal growth.
Deficiency: Nutritional macrocytic anemia.

Choline

A member of the Vitamin B Complex family. One of the "Lipotropic Factors."
Natural Sources: Egg yolks, brain, heart, green leafy vegetables and legumes, yeast, liver and wheat germ.
Functions: Regulates function of liver; necessary for normal fat metabolism. Minimizes excessive deposits of fat in liver.
Deficiency: May result in cirrhosis and fatty degeneration of liver, hardening of the arteries.

Inositol

Another member of the B Complex family.
Natural Sources: Fruits, nuts, whole grains, milk, meat, yeast.
Functions: Similar to that of Choline.
Deficiency: Similar to that of Choline.

Vitamin F

Unsaturated fatty acids, Linoleic Acid, and Linolenic Acids.
Natural Sources: Vegetable oils such as soybean, peanut, safflower, cottonseed, corn, and linseed.
Functions: A growth-promoting factor; necessary for

healthy skin, hair and glands. Promotes the availability of calcium to the cells. Now considered to be important in lowering blood cholesterol and in combatting heart disease.
Deficiency: May lead to skin disorders such as eczema.

Methionine

dl-Methionine. One of the essential Amino Acids.
Natural Sources: Meat, eggs, fish, milk, cheese.
Functions: Building new body tissue; helps to remove fat from liver.
Deficiency: May lead to fatty degeneration and cirrhosis of liver.

Biotin

One of the newly discovered members of the B Complex family.
Natural Sources: Yeast. Present in minute quantities in every living cell.
Functions: Growth-promoting factor. Possibly related to metabolism of fats and in the conversion of certain amino acids.
Deficiency: May lead to extreme exhaustion, drowsiness, muscle pains, and loss of appetite; also a type of anemia complicated by a skin disease.

Lysine

L-Lysine Monohydrochloride. One of the essential Amino Acids.
Natural Sources: Meat, eggs, fish, milk, cheese.
Functions: Building new body tissue and also vital substances such as antibodies, hormones, enzymes, and body cells.
Deficiency: Not definitely known yet.

Vitamin P

Citrus Bioflavanoids, Bioflavanoid Complex, Hesperidin.
Natural Sources: Peels and pulp of citrus fruit, especially lemon.
Functions: Strengthens walls of capillaries. Prevents Vitamin C from being destroyed in body by oxidation. Beneficial in hypertension. Reported to help build resistance in infections and colds.
Deficiency: Capillary fragility. Appearance of purplish spots on skin.

Rutin

Natural Sources: Buckwheat.
Functions: Similar to that of Vitamin P.
Deficiency: Similar to that of Vitamin P.

Paba

Para-Amino-Benzoic Acid. Belongs to the B Complex group.
Natural Sources: Yeast.
Functions: A growth-promoting factor, possibly in conjunction with Folic Acid. In experimental tests on animals, this vitamin when omitted from foods caused hair to turn white. When restored to the diet, the white hair turned black.
Deficiency: May cause extreme fatigue, eczema, anemia.

The Important Minerals

Calcium: Builds and maintains bones and teeth; helps blood to clot; aids vitality and endurance; regulates heart rhythm.

Cobalt: Stimulant to production of red blood cells; component of Vitamin B-12; necessary for normal growth and appetite.

Copper: Necessary for absorption and utilization of iron; formation of red blood cells.

Fluorine: May decrease incidence of dental caries.

Iodine: Necessary for proper function of thyroid gland; essential for proper growth, energy, and metabolism.

Iron: Required in manufacture of hemoglobin; helps carry oxygen in the blood.

Magnesium: Necessary for calcium and Vitamin C metabolism; essential for normal functioning of nervous and muscular system.

Manganese: Activates various enzymes and other minerals; related to proper utilization of Vitamins B-1 and E.

Molybdenum: Associated with carbohydrate metabolism.

Phosphorus: Needed for normal bone and tooth structure. Interrelated with action of calcium and Vitamin D.

Potassium: Necessary for normal muscle tone, nerves, heart action, and enzyme reactions.

Sulfur: Vital to good skin, hair, and nails.

Zinc: Helps normal tissue function, protein, and carbohydrate metabolism.

Sleep

All living things require periods of repose alternating with periods of activity. Sound, restful, and sufficient sleep is absolutely essential for a strong, healthy body. Sleep is caused by body fatigue acting on the nervous system, so it is obvious that the health of the nervous system cannot be maintained without regular sleep.

Sleep is just as important as food and drink. It is only during sleep that the nerve cells can accumulate energy. The result of insufficient sleep is a gradual reduction of energy until the nervous system becomes exhausted and the health undermined.

We are re-created when we sleep. Rest restores energy which has been consumed in work or physical activity. Every hour of rest before midnight saves vitality. Lack of sufficient sleep lessens our prospects for continued youthfulness and a long useful life.

The amount of sleep required by people varies according to age, sex, and habits. As a rule, seven to eight hours' sleep is about right for the normal adult. Young people (under 21 years of age) should get nine to ten hours' sleep.

In conclusion, it may be said that the general remedies for sleeplessness are actual work in the open air, a moderate amount of bodily exercise, freedom from worry and anxiety, a warm bath before going to bed if necessary, and sleeping in a well-ventilated room.

Sun Baths

Sunlight is essential for improving general health and building strong bodies and abundant vitality. Everyone looking for health and physical perfection should receive the influence of the sun's rays in the open air whenever possible. The quickest way to do this is to take a sun bath. Remember that a sun bath taken through glass loses a large amount of its value because the ultraviolet rays, which are of great importance in light therapeutics, cannot penetrate glass unless a special type of glass is used.

The rays of the sun stimulate all the functions of the body. Digestion and nutrition are improved, circulation of the blood and lymph is hastened, skin elimination is increased, and morbid tissue is broken down. The hemoglobin and red blood cells are materially increased.

The first sun bath should not last more than ten minutes, and this can be increased gradually each day until you are able to remain in the sun for from one to two hours. If remaining in the sun tends to cause headaches, a towel (dampened in cold water) may be placed around and over your head while taking the sun bath. This will also preclude any possibility of sunstroke. On the other hand, if you feel weak the following day, or have a slight fever or blistering of the skin, it is an indication that the sun bath is being overdone.

Remember that blondes, redheads, and fair-skinned persons are inclined to burn instead of tan because their skin has less protective pigment than that of darker-skinned people. These people should proceed very carefully with their sun baths.

If you cannot take a real sun bath, then you should spend as much time as possible out of doors in the sunlight as this will mean a greater measure of health, strength, and energy.

Get Outdoors and Live

In order to live in every sense of the word, you must become a part of the great outdoors. Outdoor living adds to one's vitality and vigor. It increases one's energies and enthusiasm for life.

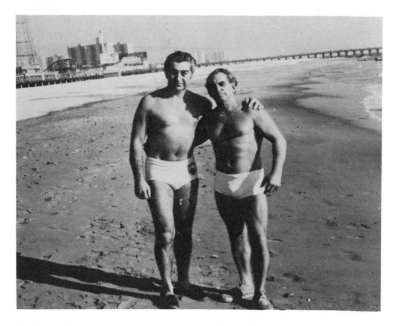

During the season when most people stay at home, Vic Boff (58) and his training partner Joe Rollino (63) enjoy the cold winter weather at Coney Island, New York. "Put wintertime back into your life. Come to this great empty beach and enjoy its challenge, its fun and tranquility. Its a great time of year and a great way of life."

202

A great many of us spend the largest part of our lives in close, badly ventilated, overheated houses. While we no longer live in treetops or in caves, there is no reason we can't make a healthy effort to get out of doors as much as possible. If there is any hobby that is worthwhile, it is one that takes us out of doors.

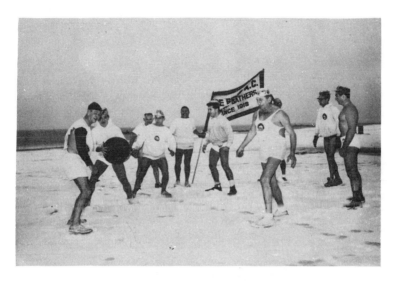

The world-famous Iceberg Athletic Club celebrates New Year's Day at the beach with a vigorous game of medicine ball and swimming in the icy Atlantic Ocean. Note Vic Boff without a shirt at the extreme right of the picture.

There are any number of outdoor sports or activities. We can compete with the elements to work off our pent-up aggressions or frustrations, try to outwit nature to improve our self-confidence, or simply enjoy being in the open air away from the artificial lives we are sometimes forced to live due to the exigencies of our time. Walking, hiking, camping, swimming, tennis, handball, cycling, and many other activities can be universally recommended for both sexes and all ages.

You don't have to be a champion at every activity. The

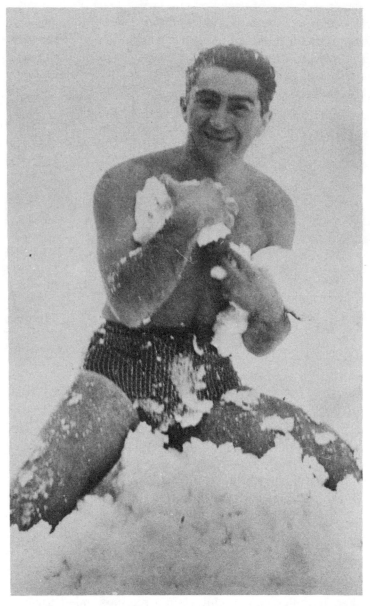

Vic Boff prepares for his swim by taking a snow bath.

idea is simply to *be* active and enthusiastic about whatever you do. Even if you are only a "dud" instead of a champion, it is better to play and be active in some outdoor effort in order to obtain the maximum amount of fun and fitness. That's what counts. For those who are less rugged, but who are all the more in need of open-air exercises for that reason, there is a great variety of nonstrenuous pastimes such as walking, hiking, cycling, and swimming, which can be enjoyed just for fun. The nature of the exercise does not matter, as long as there is a natural stimulation of all bodily processes, i.e., breathing, circulation, etc., without straining. Therefore, get out of doors and find some exercise or activity that appeals to you; an outdoor activity which will regularly take you away from the confinement of modern indoor living. You will enjoy life more, think more clearly and quickly, and your whole attitude toward life will be brighter and more discerning, and this will make you more capable of coping with the problems of day-to-day living.

I love the outdoor life. During the cold winter months, I spend my weekends at the beach, regardless of weather conditions, bathing in the icy waters of the Atlantic Ocean, running along the beach, playing medicine ball with members of the world-famous Iceberg Athletic Club. Look at the photographs, and you will understand my enthusiasm for this type of activity. While I do not recommend this type of rugged outdoor activity for the average person, I believe that most individuals can take advantage of the beach during the cold winter months by dressing comfortably, walking and jogging along the water's edge, and breathing in the healthful, pure, salt air.

If you are an outdoor man or woman, you will be able to side-step sickness, think better, eat better, sleep soundly, and feel full of the zest for living. If you want the abundant vitality which can be obtained through the open-air life, spend as much time as possible out of doors.

Use Your Time Wisely
for Bodybuilding Success

Time is one of the most valuable possessions of modern life, perhaps the most valuable. It can never be replaced. Once wasted it is gone forever. There are just so many hours in each week, and so many weeks in each year. If you invest those hours and weeks wisely, in a properly arranged course of exercise, you can build a body of muscular power and beauty that will increase your life span. If you waste it, you are not only shortening your life, but are wilfully wasting something that all the money in the world cannot buy—a strong and healthy body.

I will not attempt to tell you how much time should be spent with any type of exercise program or system. Rather, I will try to explain the meaning of time in its relationship to your life and your training, so that you will realize that this important factor cannot be overemphasized.

The bodybuilder has so much time and no more which he can devote to his training periods. Our modern, fast life has placed limitations on the use of our time. Therefore, we have to become efficiency experts in our expenditure of it. We should not be interested in how long it takes to perform an exercise or the length of time involved in finishing the workout, we should perform each and every exercise in full detail—aiming for perfection of perform- ance throughout its execution. Remember that every minute you save by properly applied scientific movement is a minute added to your life. These minutes add up to hours, days, and even years.

Applying a system to your bodybuilding program simplifies it and makes for greater progress. Working methodically, almost twice as much exercise can be performed in the same amount of time as when there isn't any system. A definite order, or plan, will help to make your bodybuilding program much more efficient, enjoyable, practical, and successful.

In starting your exercise schedule you must have a foundation program to begin with, regardless of the type of physique you have, otherwise you may be wasting your effort. From this preliminary toning stage of conditioning, progressively graduate your bodybuilding through various stages. At all times your degree of strength should be used in accordance with your bodily needs. Each series of exercise will provide a new or increased resistance to comply with the growing demands of improved physical efficiency and increased strength. Your muscles will be stimulated to healthy growth. The exercises must be graduated to enable you to control the degree of muscular growth and strength. You can stop at any stage of development deemed sufficient, or continue the scale of progression until you reach the limit of which your body is naturally capable. This is the only method to employ. It is the fastest, safest, and best.

Many bodybuilders are concerned about what time is best to work out. I have found that the evening hours are the best and most practical time to exercise. Of course, exercise should take place not less than two hours after the last meal, to give the digestion a chance. At the end of the working day the body is more responsive and mobile. It is charged with fatigue toxins. The purging processes of the blood stream are aided by the exercises and this allows the body to function more healthfully during the hours of sleep.

Exercising immediately on arising is too sudden a change for the organism. The organic tone of the body is lowered during sleep and the mobilizing of the physical forces upon awaking is too sudden a change for the body's responsive powers. Bending and stretching movements with some deep breathing exercises are helpful, but the developing movements are not recommended on arising.

Time itself has many angles attached to it. Generally, we find either haste or procrastination. The former fits the old proverb of making waste. The latter is truly known as the thief of time. Both are common faults of the unsuccessful bodybuilder. Eliminate these personality imperfections and you will turn failure into success.

The first time we try to do something which is new to us, we often find it a bit difficult. This is true about a new job, a new study, or any other new undertaking. But after the first attempt it becomes easier, and it continues to do so after each effort. You will find this to be true of your bodybuilding exercises. After the first few weeks you will be amazed at the ease with which you can master each new lesson. New exercises, which seemed difficult only because they were new, will soon become old friends. This is particularly true if you aim high, and try to perfect your performance with a minimum waste of time.

Now, if you are the type of person who chooses to skip an exercise session, or the type who says he hasn't the time for exercise, to justify a weakness or laziness, then you may as well take your place along with the other life failures. However, if you just can't find the time to carry out your planned bodybuilding program due to inefficiency in the management of your time, I suggest that you carefully analyze your daily living plan. In this way you will find the leaks and gaps delaying your efforts. With thoughtful planning, you can systematize your time, which will allow you to carry out your exercise schedule. Then you can say, "I have put living on a profitable basis, just as if I were in business." The all-important difference is that you are dealing in wealths of health and strength.

In order to eliminate your time waste, the following suggestions may prove helpful:

1. Learn what you are doing that is unnecessary, and which can therefore be omitted.

2. Find out two or three things that you do at separate times, which can be done and combined at the same time to save motions.

3. Analyze the plan you are using for your full day's activity, so that it is well balanced with work, study, recreation, and bodybuilding.

If you make a weekly record and study it carefully you will be amazed at your findings. You will become an efficiency expert in the successful administration of your own time.

Think it over carefully, and arrange your time so that you will have plenty of it to carry out a complete program of progressive exercise training which will enrich your life with health and strength, making it happier and certainly more useful and successful.

The Tools for
Physical Fitness

Walking, hiking, jogging, running, swimming, skating, cycling, and rope-skipping are excellent supplemental health and fitness exercises and activities that can be added to your bodybuilding program.

There are many excellent home exercising appliances that can be purchased and used with great benefit in your fitness and exercise schedules, including:

Adjustable Barbell and Dumbbell combination sets for the exercises outlined throughout this book.

Aluminum or Iron Health Shoes, a wonderful appliance for developing strong and shapely legs.

Chest Pulls, made with spring or rubber cables. An excellent apparatus for upper body development.

Incline Board, also known as abdominal or slant board. Great for the abdominal and waist-trimming exercises.

Doorway Gym Bar, an adjustable appliance that fits in most doorways. Excellent for stretching, isometric, and upper body exercises.

Stationary Bikes and Treadmills on which you can pedal or walk your way to a slimmer, firmer figure without leaving home. Excellent for all members of the family.

The Multi-Lift Exerciser, which can be used as an all-around fitness, body, and strength builder. Provides a progressive, graduated system of body culture that is simple, safe, and sure. Can be adapted equally well to the weakest individual and to the strongest athlete.

210

Visit the sporting goods department at your favorite store. Ask to see the complete exercise line.

For any additional information, address inquiries to:

Vic Boff

92 Cathedral Station,

New York, N.Y. 10025

Index

Abdomen, 68–69
  exercising, proper position for,
  71–72
Abdominal exercises, 73–81
  advanced, 81–85
Achilles tendon, 88
Adam's apple, 130
Arm exercises, 148–165
Arm muscles, 147

Backbone, 54
Back exercises, 112–128
Barbell exercises, 163–165
Biceps, 88, 147
  exercises, 150–153
Bodybuilding, natural methods
  of, 6
  scheduling time for, 206–209
Breathing, proper, 9–13
  development, 57
  efficient, 21–22
Breastbone, 54
Breastplate (pectoral) muscles,
  55–56

Calisthenics, 5–6
Carbohydrates, 183–184
Carotid arteries, 131
Cervical vertebrae, 130–131
Chest, 52–59
  exercises without apparatus,
  59–60
  exercises with apparatus, 61–
  67
  increasing size of, 55
Clavical stage, of breathing, 57

Diaphragm stage, of breathing,
  57
Dorsal vertebrae, 54
Dumbbells, 22–23
  exercises with, 154–165

Esophagus, 131
Evacuation, stimulating natural
  process of, 25–27
Exercises
  abdominal, 73–81
  arm, 148–165
  back, 112–128
  barbell, 163–165
  biceps, 150–153
  chest, 59–67
  dumbbells, 154–165
  foot, 163–174
  forearm, 153–154
  hip joints, 34–39
  leg, 39–42, 88–102
  method of, 48–51
  neck, 134–144
  shoulders, 42–47
  spine, 30–34, 112–128
  stretching, 166–170
  triceps, 148–150
  vitality-building, 29–47
  waist, 30–34

Fats, 184–185
Fitzsimmons, Bob, 56
Foot exercises, 173–174

Hernia, 57
Hip exercises, 34–39

Iceberg Athletic Club, 203
Intercostal muscles, 54
Intercostal stage of breathing, 57
Internal massage, 24–25

Jugular veins, 131

Larynx, 131
Latissimi dorsi muscles, 58, 114
Latissimus muscles, 53
Legs
    exercises for, 29–42, 88–109
    muscles of, 87–88
Lumbago, 111
Lumbar region, 111, 115
    toning, 28–30

Minerals, 187, 197–198
Mineral-vitamin chart, 190–198
Muscular stimulation, 71
Muscles, 48, 175–179

Natural methods of bodybuilding,
    6
Neck
    coordinating movements of,
    136–137
    exercises, 135–144
    lower joint of, 137
    muscles, 130–131
    strength, 132
Nutrition planning, 188–189

Pectoral muscles, 54, 55–56
Pelvic area, limbering, 27–28
Pelvis, 111
Physical Culture magazine, 175
Physical fitness tools, 210
Posture, 14–18
Prolapse, 57
Proteins, 183

Quadriceps femoris muscles, 87,
    88

Rectus abdominis muscles, 69
Rectus femoris muscles, 88
Ribs, 54

Roughage, 187–188

Sacral region, toning, 28–30
Sartorius muscles, 88
Sciatic nerve, 172
Serratus magnus muscles, 54, 56–
    57
Shopping for health, 189–190
Shoulder exercises, 42–47
Sleep, amount required, 199
Small of back, toning, 28–30
Soleus muscle, 88
Sphincter, 69
Spinal column exercises, 30–34
Spine
    exercises for, 112–128
    how thrown out of alignment,
    112
Spinae erector muscles, 114
Splenius capitas muscle, 134
Splenius cervicis muscle, 134
Splenius muscle, 134
Sternocleidomastoid muscle, 132,
    133
Sternum, 54
Stomach distension, 57
Stretching exercises, 166–170
    advanced, 170–171
Sun bathing, 200–201

Tensor fascia lata muscle, 88
Thoracic vertebrae, 54
Thorax, 54
Toning, 5–7
Tools for physical fitness, 210
Trachea, 131
Trapezius muscles, 58, 114, 132,
    134
Triceps muscle, 147
    exercises for, 148–150

Vastus internus muscle, 87
Vertebrae, 111
Vitamins, 185–186, 190–197

Waistline, 68
    exercises for, 30–34
Water, 187